Education for Gerontic Nursing

EDUCATION FOR GERONTIC NURSING

Laurie M. Gunter, R.N., Ph.D.
Carmen A. Estes, R.N., Ph.D.

Springer Publishing Company
New York

Copyright © 1979 by Springer Publishing Company, Inc.

All rights reserved

No part of this publication may be reproduced, stored in a retrieval system, or transmitted, in any form or by any means, electronic, mechanical, photocopying, recording, or otherwise, without the prior permission of Springer Publishing Company, Inc.

Springer Publishing Company, Inc.
200 Park Avenue South
New York, N.Y. 10003

79 80 81 82 83 / 10 9 8 7 6 5 4 3 2 1

Library of Congress Cataloging in Publication Data

Gunter, Laurie M   1922–
   Education for gerontic nursing.

  (Springer series on the teaching of nursing; v. 5)
  Bibliography: p.
  Includes index.
  1. Geriatric nursing—Study and teaching.   I. Estes, Carmen A., joint author.   II. Title.   III. Series.
RC954.G85   610.73'65   78-10472
ISBN 0-8261-2450-X
ISBN 0-8261-2451-8 pbk.

Printed in the United States of America

Contents

Preface   vii
1. Introduction   1
2. Problems and Issues in the Care of the Aging   15
3. The Study and Practice of Nursing the Aged   27
4. Preparing the Nurse's Aide for Gerontic Nursing   41
5. Preparing the Licensed Practical Nurse for Gerontic Nursing   53
6. Undergraduate Education in Gerontic Nursing   65
7. Graduate Education in Gerontic Nursing   81
8. Preparing the Geriatric Nurse Practitioner   139
9. Continuing Education in Gerontic Nursing   147

Appendixes
   A. A Guide to Content Analysis for Computer-based Nursing Courses   165
   B. A Course Model for Computer-based Instruction   169
   C. A Course Outline for Gerontic Nursing   181
   D. A Sample of a Short-term Training Program   183

Bibliography   193

Index   205

Preface

The purpose of this book is to provide a conceptual framework, delineation, and definition for a field of nursing practice and research pertaining to the nursing care of the elderly; to set forth a list of assumptions general to this area of specialization in nursing, along with assumptions specific to each of five levels of nursing practice; to describe the curricular implications of the assumptions, the competencies expected at each of the five practice levels, and where appropriate, a curriculum framework; to organize some of the existing knowledge and resources and make them available in a usable and readily accessible form; and to stimulate the development of additional knowledge through utilization of research methods.

The objectives are: (1) to provide an overview of the current state of the art in practice, education, and research in the nursing care of the elderly; (2) to provide nursing educators in nursing schools and in-service education personnel in hospitals, nursing homes, home nursing programs, and long-term care facilities with guidelines for curriculum structure and educational resources for five levels of nursing personnel; and (3) to formulate long-range trends, needs, and directions for practice, education, and research in the nursing care of the elderly, and to make recommendations and suggestions for action where feasible.

Education for Gerontic Nursing was prepared with support from Nursing Special Project Grant number 5 D10 NU 0 1160–03, formerly 03D–005340, U.S. Department of Health, Education and Welfare, Bureau of Health Manpower Education, Division of Nursing.

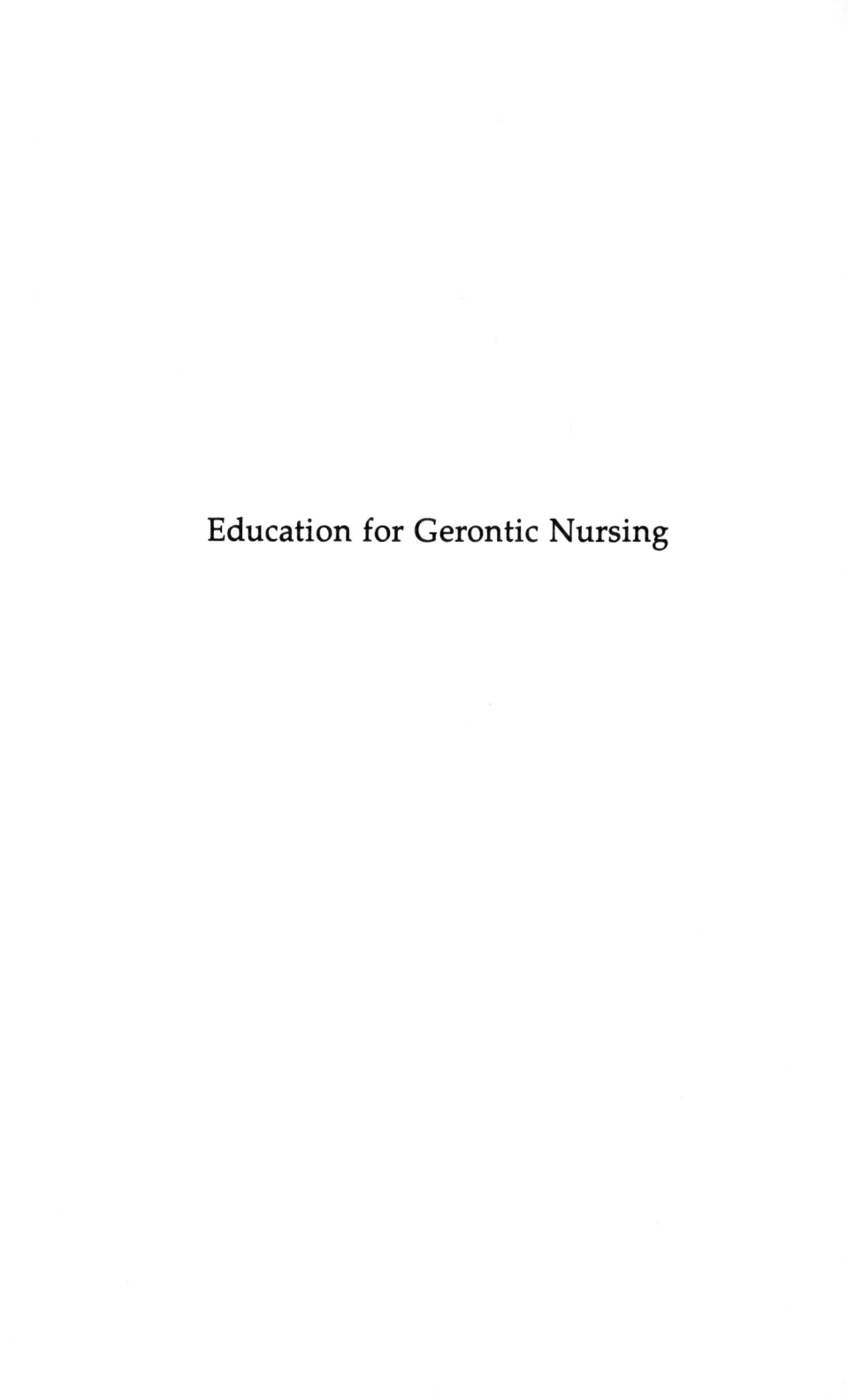

Education for Gerontic Nursing

1
Introduction

The provision of adequate health care for the advanced in age is one of the more pressing issues in our society today. Life expectancy has been extended from an average of 47 years in the early 1900s to an average of more than 70 years in 1970 and is still increasing. The problems of the aged are multiple and involve money, health, and meaningful roles in society. Ten percent of the population are 65 years of age or over, and it is expected that by the end of this century there will be 25 million Americans over 65 and that the proportion of those over 75 will have increased significantly. The 10 percent of our population who are over 65 occupy 25 percent of the available hospital beds and account for 25 percent of the national cost of medical care. In addition, there are approximately 23,000 nursing homes containing over a million beds in the United States. We now have more nursing-home beds than hospital beds.

Despite these statistics and the fact that only 4 percent of old people are living in institutions, the quality of care and custodial services provided in some instances are considered a national disgrace, to be utilized only by those disabled whose resources have been depleted.

While the greater majority of old people are not institutionalized, most of them could benefit from health care which includes counseling, teaching, and advising about how to maintain health and vigor. Their health care should also include care in preventing complications as well as providing restorative and rehabilitative services and supporting home care services that will allow them to remain in their family homes and communities.[1]

Although in the past modern science has succeeded in increasing longevity, few adequate and accessible programs were developed in any of the care professions to deal specifically with the developing health needs of the geriatric person. No orderly, systematic educational experiences designed to prepare care personnel to deal with the health and/or illness needs of this population group were available. People were placed in institutions as a means of meeting their health care needs, as well as the personal crises of aging. The assumption has often been made, perhaps erroneously, that elderly persons should be institutionalized, grouped in housing centers with others of similar age, and cared for as health and living problems developed. In light of current thinking and emphasis on health needs of different age groups in society, haphazard planning is no longer appropriate. Further, the majority of the aging population consists of the healthy aged; therefore, gerontic nursing care should include emphasis on health promotion and maintenance.

A Composite Educational Program for Geriatric Nursing

Nursing, which accounts for the largest number of workers in the health professions, has a special responsibility for health promotion activities, including teaching, advising, counseling, and demonstrating health care measures. Since many gerontological behaviors are the result of environmental deprivation, it is only logical that nursing should also become involved as a change agent in designing, planning, and implementing healthful environments for the aged.

The project "Composite Educational Program for Geriatric Nursing" was proposed to increase the supply of adequately trained nursing personnel to meet the health and nursing care needs of this age group. (The term "program" as used in this application refers to a geriatric emphasis within existing nursing programs.) The project was carried out under Title II of the Health Manpower Act of 1968 (P.L. 90-490). This act provided for the continuation and broadening of the special projects for improvement in nurse training under the Nurse Training Act of 1964 (P.L. 88-581, Title VIII, Nurse Training), which authorized grants to schools of nursing to assist them in meeting additional costs of projects designed to strengthen, improve, or expand programs to teach and train nurses. The authority for special project grants was extended for three years by the Nurse Training Act of 1971 (P.L. 92-158).[2] Included in the purposes of special project grants, as specified in Section 805(a) of the Act, was one to develop training programs and to train personnel for new roles, types, or levels of nursing, including programs for the training of pediatric and other types of nurse practitioners.

The intent of the project was to help nursing fulfill its special responsibility to the aged through a comprehensive program incorporating resident instruction (undergraduate and graduate education); continuing education-community services; and research emanating from an educational program designed specifically for the purpose of providing composite preparation, community services, and research directed toward improved geriatric care in homes, communities, and institutions.

Objectives

The project focussed on the problem of defining levels of preparation, and what kinds of materials and learning experiences are appropriate for preparing personnel at various levels. The care personnel were specified at five levels:

1. Level I: on-the-job training (nurse's aide)
2. Level II: vocational education (licensed practical nurse)

3. Level III: post high school and undergraduate baccalaureate education (registered nurse)
4. Level IV: graduate education at the master's degree level
5. Level V: graduate education at the doctoral level

The major objectives of the project were to determine the kinds of materials and learning experiences appropriate for preparing personnel for the five levels and to develop instructional methods and materials that could be utilized in teaching appropriate content to personnel in the five levels.

The specific objectives of the project were to:

1. Design courses including objectives, content, learning experiences, and evaluation of various curriculums and continuing education programs
2. Develop instructional materials for use in teaching programs related to professional nursing roles and other nursing personnel providing care for the aged
3. Implement courses, workshops, seminars, and the evaluation of outcomes of such activities
4. Publish results

The educational materials and experiences were designed to include the following personnel.

Students in a baccalaureate nursing program who require basic knowledge and skills in the nursing care of the elderly, and those who need additional knowledge and skills because they have chosen to prepare for work in nursing settings which provide care to the elderly. The latter group of students would begin an elective in this specialized area of nursing practice.

Registered nurses graduating from diploma and associate degree programs who need sufficient basic preparation to understand the aging process, the social problems accompanying the aging process, and the health care problems, as well as the basic skills for carrying out the restorative, preventive, and maintenance aspects of nursing care.

Registered nurses, preferably with a baccalaureate or higher degree, who assume responsibility for staff development in facilities designed for long-term care. The materials developed for

Levels I and II were to be used in preparing nurses for this function.

Registered nurses preparing for the gerontic nurse practitioner role who require preparation for providing primary health care for older patients in organized ambulatory and home care service agencies.

Graduate students in nursing preparing for the adult health and aging specialist role who require preparation for conducting such health care services for the aged as counseling, advising, teaching, and referral and follow-up in community-based facilities.

Graduate students in nursing preparing for the role of gerontic nurse specialist or long-term care specialist who require preparation for maintaining a stable state in chronically ill patients such as those in nursing homes or other institutions for long-term care, and for assessing changes in conditions, planning nursing care, preventing complications, instituting rehabilitative measures, and consulting with the physician as changes in conditions necessitate changes in the medically prescribed therapeutic regimes.

Nursing administrators of long-term care facilities.

Graduate students in nursing seeking preparation at the doctoral level for teaching and research in adult development and aging and adult health and aging.

Table 1-1 delineates plans for the composite educational program and includes the level, target population, previous educational background, educational mechanism, and the proposed content in aging by level. Table 1-2 summarizes the educational levels and roles in gerontic nursing defined in the project.

Guides to Program Development

For the purpose of the Composite Educational Program certain general assumptions were set forth by the project staff:

1. The American population is an aging population.
2. Aging persons use a disproportionate share of the available health services.
3. The health care system in American society has not provided accessible and adequate services for older Americans.

Table 1-1.
Plans for the Composite Preparation of Nursing Personnel for Care of Geriatric Patients and Persons Advanced in Age

Levels	Target Population	Educational Background	Educational Mechanism	Proposed Content in Aging
I* On-the-job Training	Aides and technicians	None	Staff development—in-service, managed and taught by a registered nurse	1. Basic nursing care skills 2. Normal aging process 3. Elementary rehabilitation nursing care skills 4. Human relations skills with emphasis on relating to older people
II* Vocational	Licensed practical nurses	Course for licensure—usually one year	Staff development—in-service, managed and taught by a registered nurse	1. Introductory aspects of the social psychological, and physical aspects of aging 2. Selected rehabilitation nursing skills 3. Nursing care of the terminally ill and dying

III A Basic professional	Nursing students (generic level)	Fundamentals of nursing course	Formal courses including theory and clinical practice; elective courses for those wishing to begin specialization in the nursing care of the elderly	1. Physiological, psychological, and sociological aspects of aging 2. Common health problems of the aged 3. Nursing process focused on the care of the elderly and including rehabilitation 4. Drug therapy and interaction
III B Professional	Registered nurses	Basic nursing program—diploma, associate, or baccalaureate degree	Continuing education	Same as above with modifications
III C Gerontic Nurse Practitioner	Students with advanced standing in baccalaureate program or registered nurses; students in master's level who wish to develop selected skills	Theory and skills of III A or III B	Formal courses including theory and practice	1. Family and community relationships 2. Methods of health assessment 3. Management of the chronically ill aged based on advanced knowledge, i.e., pathology, drug management, and rehabilitation

Table 1-1. (*continued*)

Levels	Target Population	Educational Background	Educational Mechanism	Proposed Content in Aging
III D In-service educators	Registered nurses	Theory and skills of Levels III A or III B	Continuing education	Content derived from above for: 1. Teaching/learning strategies 2. Design of learning modules 3. Evaluation and assessment of learner performance 4. Practicum in staff development
IV Advanced/Master's level IV A Specialist in gerontic nursing	Registered nurses	Baccalaureate degree in nursing	Formal courses leading to a master's degree, including theory and practice	1. Advanced work in the clinical management of geriatric patients 2. Counseling techniques for working with patients and their families 3. Therapeutic management of nursing environments 4. Management of psychopathology in the aged

			5. Planning and evaluation of the utilization of nursing resources
6. Pharmacological principles for drug administration in the elderly
IV B
Specialist in adult health and aging	Registered nurse	Baccalaureate degree in nursing	Formal courses leading to a master's degree, including theory and practice	1. Advanced work in teaching and advising the elderly and planning educational programs
2. As above in IV A
3. Development and utilization of community resources
4. Preparation for recognition of physical and mental pathologic changes, referral to appropriate agencies
5. Planning and evaluation of community health programs
6. As above in IV A
7. Provision of maintenance care and rehabilitation of elderly living in the community

Table 1-1. (continued)

Levels	Target Population	Educational Background	Educational Mechanism	Proposed Content in Aging
IV C Administrator of nursing service in long-term care facilities	Registered nurses	Baccalaureate degree in nursing	Formal courses leading to a master's degree, including theory and practice	As in IV A above, plus courses in nursing home administration, including personnel management and knowledge of state and federal regulalations in lieu of IV A 1 and IV A 4
V Graduate at doctoral level Nurse scientist/ gerontologist	Registered nurses	Graduate education at the master's level—preparation as a gerontic nursing specialist or specialist in adult health and aging	College or university program at doctoral level (human development and family studies and other areas)	1. Courses and seminars in theories of aging and development, and nursing care 2. Research methodology with emphasis on nursing gerontology

*Indirect training program through preparation of registered nurses for in-service education or staff development.

Table 1-2.
Educational Levels and Roles in Gerontic Nursing

Levels	End Product
Level I: on-the-job training	Technicians and aides in institutions
	Home health aides
Level II: vocational education	Licensed practical nurses in institutional care services
	Lincensed practical nurses in home health agencies
*Level III: registered nurse education	Registered nurses as staff nurses in institutional settings
a. generic level	Staff nurses in community and home health services
b. post-registered nurse level	Nurse practitioners in ambulatory services
	In-service educators
*Level IV: graduate education at the master's degree level	Geriatric nursing specialists
	Adult health and aging specialists
	Nurse administrators in long-term care institutions
*Level V: graduate education at the doctoral level	Teachers and researchers in gerontology and geriatric nursing/gerontologists

*Levels for which educational materials have been prepared or described.

4. A great majority of the aging population consists of the healthy aged, hence comprehensive gerontic nursing care should include emphasis on health promotion and maintenance.

5. Health promotion services need to be greatly expanded and professional nurses should assume major responsibility for health promotion activities.

6. Increasingly, gerontological behaviors are shown to be mostly a consequence of environmental deprivations; therefore, nurses should become involved as change agents in designing, planning, and implementing healthful environments for the old.

7. Only 4 percent of the aged population reside in institutions but the poor quality of care they receive in many instances is a major concern of professional nurses as well as patients and their families.

8. Much of the institutional care of the aged is and will be given by nonprofessional nursing personnel who need inservice preparation by professional nurses trained for this task.

9. In 1966, the American Nurses' Association recognized geriatrics as a specialty area by establishing the Geriatric Division of Nursing Practice; therefore, basic professional education for nurses should provide a knowledge base that would enable the beginning practitioner to provide comprehensive and therapeutic nursing care to the middle-aged and elderly. Specialization at the graduate level is necessary to provide the socialization and knowledge necessary for interdisciplinary team work and leadership necessary to fulfill nursing's responsibility to the elderly.

10. Emphasis on research and clinical studies is needed to improve the quality of nursing care and should become an important component of the composite educational program.

Some guidelines were established for selecting and developing instruction units and materials. These units and materials should present a representative and realistic view of aging devoid, insofar as possible, of positive and negative stereotypes and support the general belief or philosophy that aging is a normal process with individual variability, including a balance of emphasis on such features as function and dysfunction, dependence and independence. In addition, it was felt important that the units and materials be up-to-date and accurate; identify sources and resources; be prepared in a format suitable for publication; and allow for evaluation.

Recommendations for Geronic Nursing Education

During the course of the project we considered the educational needs of five levels of nursing personnel, beginning with the aide and going to the licensed practical nurse, the registered nurse, the specialist in nursing with master's degree preparation, and the specialist with preparation for the doctoral degree. We began to see clearly how some of the educational problems prevalent today arose out of the misuse of personnel, particularly the nurse's aide, in facilities designed for persons requiring long-term care. We came to the following conclusions. First, we must make explicit the fact that the nurse's aide is not a nurse. The nurse's aide is or should be prepared to assist the nurse with delegated tasks, usually those limited to the personal care of patients who have some deficit or decrement in their self-maintenance skills. Second, there are two licensed practitioners in nursing—the licensed practical nurse and the registered nurse. We propose to provide basic in-service education, staff development, and continuing education for these two levels of nursing together. Inasmuch as the licensed practical nurse program is usually limited to 9 to 12 months, it was thought best not to attempt to tamper with this particular curriculum but to provide preparation for the nursing care of the elderly through informal modalities. In terms of the baccalaureate degree program which nursing envisions as becoming the basic professional program for the profession of nursing, we recommend the inclusion of gerontic nursing content, as is done with four other divisions of nursing practices—medical-surgical, maternal-child, community health, and psychiatric-mental health. This would be in keeping with the structural organization of the American Nurses' Association (ANA), and certainly in support of the need for health care among the elderly population, which probably supercedes that of any other age group in demand. We emphasize the need for nursing specialization at the master's level and for doctoral preparation as the preparation for research in nursing. Further, we emphasize the necessity to draw heavily on the content from gerontology and studies of aging; to consider the area of gerontic nursing as deriving from the interaction of health status and aging; and to acknowledge that nursing research into the problems of the elderly may require the use of concepts and methods from several disciplines including nursing. Finally, we are impressed with the vast literature and resources available to be used in developing educational programs and in scientific studies. The need for synthesizing this knowledge, translating it into principles and guides, and making applications to nursing practice presents a tremendous challenge to gerontic nurses.

2

Problems and Issues in the Care of the Aging*

Nursing care of the aged is ageless—as is nursing in general. It began when the first old person became ill, and it will continue until human life as we know it ceases to exist. To document the long existence of our interest in caring for the elderly, we may turn to the work of Galen, a physician born in Asia Minor in 131 A.D.

> ... [T]hese and other things are very easy, but to take charge of an old man, safeguarding his health, is one of the most difficult; as it is also of those convalescent from disease. This latter portion of the art is called by younger physicians analepsy; and that which concerns the old man, gerontology.[1]

The concern is clearly old; what is new is the evolving science of gerontology and the evolving nursing specialization in the care of the elderly, particularly in the United States. Interest

*Reprinted from Madeleine M. Leininger, Ed. *Transcultural Nursing Care of the Elderly.* Proceedings from the Second National Transcultural Nursing Conference, Salt Lake City: University of Utah College of Nursing, 1977.

in aging and gerontology has increased in the twentieth century and has provided a favorable climate for study and research for a number of reasons. The aged have more visibility; they are retired from the work force; their numbers and proportion in the population have increased; more and more of them live in urban, industrialized areas; and the average life expectancy has increased.

In order to examine the nature of the problems and cultural issues involved in nursing care of the elderly in American society today, a framework with three components is presented: (1) old age in the context of life in society, including the responsibilities of, and the liabilities to, society as a whole for the aging population; (2) old age as a stage in human development with particular conditions, rather than merely the period of declining functions; (3) old age and cultural values in terms of who should care for the aged. These problems and issues have already been recognized and certain efforts are being made to contend with some of them. However, far more effort needs to be exerted on behalf of the elderly in the United States, especially in the area of health care delivery.

Old Age and Our Society

Society's responsibilities and liabilities for the aging population include attention to quality of life, stereotypes and misconceptions about the aging, the distribution of income, and the provision of support systems. Relevant questions confronting society today are: How can our social organization be structured so that older people may continue to remain actively involved to the extent that they desire rather than be isolated from the mainstream of life? How can we avoid delegating to the aged only those facilities and resources that are left over after the needs of other age groups have been fulfilled? How can society be structured so that older people can continue to contribute to the general welfare for as long as they wish and for as long as they can? How can we prevent their isolation and loneliness? How can we provide for their safety and welfare when they become physically frail? How can we organize activities so that they will not be ruled out of community participation? For example, with increasing years most people experience a declining ability to cope with high-density groups, traffic, crime, air pollution, and, particularly, modern modes of transportation. Will communities give the aged more consideration in planning the structure of houses, neighborhoods, streets, street lighting, and transit systems so that older people may continue to be mobile?

Quality of Life

The phrase "quality of life" means different things to different people; however, it implies concern for maintaining interest in life, zest for living, and meaningful and satisfying activities and relationships.

Robert Butler, in his Pulitzer prize winning book, *Why Survive? Being Old in America*,[2] answers the question, "What are an individual's chances for a good old age in America with satisfying final years and a dignified death?" He states that for many elderly Americans old age is a tragedy—a period of quiet despair, deprivation, desolation, and muted rage. Butler notes that this can be a consequence of the kind of life a person has led in younger years, problems in relationships with others, and the inevitable personal and physical losses which can be devastating and unbearable. However, he also points out that old age can be a tragedy for people who have had fulfilling younger years, and this is what he considers the genuine tragedy of old age in America. We have shaped a society that is extremely harsh to live in when one is old. Butler further notes that the tragedy of old age is not the fact that each of us must grow older and die but that the process of doing so has been made unnecessarily painful, humiliating, debilitating, and isolating through insensitivity, ignorance, and poverty. He says that the potentials for satisfactions in late life have been vastly underdeveloped or underexplored.

Attitudes, Stereotypes, and Myths

Agism is the stereotyping of, and discrimination against, people because they are old, just as racism is discrimination because of color and sexism is discrimination because of sex.[3] Butler describes current myths about aging.

First, it is a myth to measure age chronologically because there are great differences in the rate of physiological, psychological, and social aging from person to person.

The second myth is the myth of unproductivity. Many people believe that the old are unproductive but, in the absence of disease and social adversities, old people tend to remain productive.

Third is the myth of disengagement, which grew out of some gerontologists' views that older people choose to disengage from life, to withdraw into themselves, and to live alone or perhaps only with their peers. The fourth myth is that older people are inflexible. Butler believes that ability to change and adapt has little to do with one's age and more to do with one's lifelong character.

The fifth myth, the notion that old people are senile, or show forgetfulness, confusion, and reduced attention, is widely accepted. Butler shows that senility is a popular lay term used by doctors and the public alike. Much of the behavior lumped together as senility is treatable and often reversible.

The sixth myth—that of serenity—portrays old age as a kind of adult fairyland in which people are relatively peaceful and serene and where they can relax and enjoy the fruits of their labor after the storms of active life are over. But old people, like young people, continue to experience a full range of emotions including anger, anxiety, grief, depression, and paranoia. Butler discusses the advertising slogans that point up the myth of serenity. He states that depressive reactions are widespread, particularly in later life, and that grief is a frequent companion of old age, as is anxiety.

On the other hand, professional literature presents a negative stereotype of "old," and this negative stereotype has influenced self-concept in later life, as Brubaker and Powers note.[4] Based on their analysis of 47 such reports, several of which presented a positive stereotype, they argued that acceptance of a positive or negative stereotype by the aged is related to objective indicators of old age as well as to the subjective definition of self and self-concept.

Distribution of Income

Another very important area of concern is the distribution of income as it relates to the elderly. How can we protect older people on fixed pensions from inflationary costs and increasing taxes? Will we insist upon an escalation clause in pensions as well as in wages? Will we attempt to establish some criteria for the equitable distribution of income between the very youngest through the oldest age groups? Who will bear the burden of our increasing dependency ratio? (Dependency ratio is the ratio of the proportion of youth not yet in the work force plus the proportion of older people who have been retired from the work force to the proportion of working men and women.)

In a national survey sponsored by the Institute of Life Insurance,[5] a majority of the respondents agreed, "Most people don't have enough money to do what they want to do in retirement" (74 percent endorsed this statement fully). An overall 74 percent of the sample also said that retired people do not have enough money. (Does any age group have enough money?) We have accepted as fact that poverty is associated with aging, but Neugarten[6] states that the stereotype of the old as needy persons may be blown out of proportion since we, as professionals, tend to focus on that proportion of the elderly who have substantial problems. She reports results on a major national poll which showed that the public thinks the conditions of older persons are much more negative than older persons themselves do. For example, 60 percent of the respondents answered that most older people have a major problem with money. Yet, of the older people in this sample, only 15 percent said that money is a major problem.

Support Systems

According to a report from the "Congress on the Quality of Life—the Later Years," older people are stereotyped as "poverty-stricken, ill, and confined to institutions, abandoned by their children and other relatives, unemployed, asexual, confused, and a burden on society."[7] However, this same report shows that only 4 to 5 percent of persons over 65 live in institutions at any one time and that the "good old days" were not as good as the present day in regard to living conditions for the aged.

Other stereotypes and misconceptions exist about older people in our society and their family relationships. For example, Neugarten[8] states that older people choose to live in households separate from their children when they have the financial resources for doing so. The fact that older people tend to maintain independent households does not mean that emotionally satisfying family ties do not exist or that the old are necessarily isolated. In fact, emotionally satisfying ties may be strengthened and family conflicts lessened by independent living arrangements for older family members.

Old Age as a Stage in Human Development

Consideration of old age as a phase of human development with particular conditions rather than a period of declining functions will help determine society's response to old age. For example, if old age were seen as a stage of development, society would provide for it as such, and there would be opportunities for the older age group to continue to work toward self-actualization. There would certainly be greater acceptance of full participation of the aged in the social process. Furthermore, our ideas of health and disease would likely be affected since we tend to focus more intently on the problems of care for the small proportion of the elderly who need to be institutionalized than we do on the large proportion of the elderly who have particular strengths and experiences to share with the community as a whole.

Developmental Processes

Biologists usually define aging as the progressive loss of functional capacity as the organism reaches maturity. Increasingly, behavioral scientists view aging as a developmental continuum while admitting that there are usually cumulative losses and physical decrements correlated with aging. Their concern is with the new goals and developmental tasks the aged can achieve while making effective compensation and developing coping strategies to maintain appropriate functioning. The task, in other words, is to make life satisfying, fulfilling, and worthwhile to the end. The challenge and task have been more recently described by Butler in the phrase, "life as a work of art."[9] Butler notes that none of us knows whether we have already had the best years of our lives or whether the best are yet to come. But, he states, the greatest of human possibilities remain to the very end of life—the possibilities of love and feeling, reconciliation and resolution.

An informal survey of the faculty affiliates of the Gerontology Center at The Pennsylvania State University in 1976 pointed up the following list of concerns about the aged.

1. Many younger people perceive older people as being unable to learn (change); indeed they feel they should not try to learn (change). Many older people are convinced by younger people's perception of them. Their low self-perceptions seem to be based in part on mandatory retirement ages, often below 60 years. Older people seem to derive their images of self-worth from their jobs rather than from who they are as people.

2. A major problem in dealing with the aging and the elderly is preparing individuals psychologically and socially for what should be (but is not) the blessing of having earned respite from "productive work," and encouraging and enabling them to invest their time, energy, and abilities in self-cultivation or self-actualization.

3. Before *behavioral intervention* with the elderly and adults is undertaken, some questions should be answered: What is optimal development and who decides this? When should we intervene? Who has to agree? These questions are philosophical and ethical in nature.

Self-actualization

Do our ethics, mores, customs, and laws allow adults opportunities for self-actualization, or are the penalties too great for most people to aspire to it? For example, most middle-agers are discouraged from mid-life career changes, divorces, or change in living arrangements, particularly if these involve sexual relationships. Their grown children become greatly concerned over any changes in parental spending patterns or loving patterns and cause parents to seek psychiatric consultation or even institutionalize them. Can we develop a socialization pattern that will support self-actualization for large numbers of old persons in this society? Perhaps the major issue here is how to determine the difference between self-actualization and psychopathology in older persons who seek major changes in their life styles.

Butler[10] suggests that to avoid "lives of quiet desperation," pseudo-lives, infra-lives, and other forms of maladaptation, people need more freedom to become what they can become and what they want to become. Today, for one to make a career switch, to get off the career ladder—to make changes as a train switches tracks—is to be considered sick. Butler suggests that in some situations the more sick things a person does, the healthier he becomes.

Health and Disease

According to Busse,[11] the biological process of aging is associated with a decline of efficiency and functioning that eventually results in death. Some biologists define aging as the progressive loss of functional capacity of an organism as it reaches maturity. Others state that aging begins with the onset of differentiation, and still others do not find it possible or useful to define the aging processes.

The process of aging may be separated into primary and secondary aging. Biological processes of change are called primary aging, and are apparently controlled by heredity. These changes are inherent, inevitable, and time-related but are independent of stress, trauma, or disease. Aging does not progress at the same rate in all people. Secondary aging refers to disabilities resulting from trauma, stress, and chronic disease. The word *aged* is used arbitrarily to describe or define persons who have achieved a certain chronological age within a given population; for example, age 65. But objective changes vary widely at any particular chronological age and in different cultures, since a 40-year-old person in an underdeveloped society may be considered "old" and may have only as many years to live as a 65-year-old person in a highly developed society.

Chronic disease and secondary aging are, for all practical purposes, synonymous, since they are associated with permanent change and damage to the body. The incidence of chronic illness advances steadily with age. Busse reports that among young adults under 45 years of age, 35.3 percent of all persons have one or more chronic conditions; but 61.3 percent of persons between the ages of 45 and 54 have chronic conditions; and 78.7 percent of those 65 years and older are affected by chronic disorders.

In our society, major issues revolve around the cost, availability, and quality of health care for the whole population and what kind of national health insurance should be made available. Substantial federal funds have already been allocated for the health care of the elderly through Medicare and Medicaid. In a discussion of the problems of high costs, inadequate access to medical care, and unsatisfactory levels of health from an economic viewpoint, Fuchs stated: "For most Americans, better health is not the only, nor even most important, goal. For most Americans, more medical care is not the only, or even the most promising, route to better health."[12] Have we carefully studied what are the most important goals and desires of the aged, or have we assumed, from our vested interest as health care providers, that health is the most important goal in life?

Old Age and Cultural Values

Who should care, why should they care, and how should they care for the elderly? Answers to these questions involve attitudes that influence appropriate social roles and relationships of the family and professional caretakers, and consideration of alternatives to institutional care. In addition, the answers involve consideration of who should be taught, and what kinds of knowledge should be taught, and by whom—the elderly themselves or people from all generational groups?

Professional Caretakers

The relationship between the elderly and their family members or significant others and the quality of care provided by professionals are the crux of the problem of who should care. Are both the caring and cared-for groups affected by the general stereotype as described above, and does this affect provisions made for the care of the elderly and the quality of care provided by the caretakers?

Do we overemphasize the delivery of medical services and the prolongation of life but neglect the psychosocial aspects of life that make living worthwhile? Do we rely too much on rules and regulations to produce quality and pay too little attention to the preparation of health personnel who need to understand the process of aging and the person who ages? Can older people themselves be better prepared to maintain health, cope with disabilities, and be more independent of professional caretakers? Do we, as a society, foster sick behavior and dependency?

An issue that has scarcely been touched upon by students of geriatric nursing is what it means to a nurse to work in a geriatric facility. We need to address realistically how difficult this work is, how difficult it may be for the nurse to maintain an optimistic, cheerful demeanor when many patients have discouraging conditions, when family members are difficult to please, and when the older person himself becomes depressed and cantankerous. How do we provide the supports needed by nurses who must work from day to day in an environment that is often overladen with distress, discomfort, and disease?

Ethical problems and issues that beset professional caretakers include euthanasia, prolongation of life, and research using elderly people. Who should make the decisions about the use of expensive, life-prolonging measures? The person himself, the family, the courts, the church, or the professional caretakers?

Alternatives to Institutional Care

Decisions about provision of care for the aged when they can no longer provide for themselves, are determined by the relationships between parents, children, and grandchildren. They decide who is able and willing to provide the supports needed as alternatives to institutional care. Have we become a society that readily invests in resources for physical care but leaves many of the most advanced in age lonely and without emotional concern? When older persons have no relatives to express such concern, it must then come from the members of the community, the society in which people age. Can we develop roles and relationships to provide this kind of support?

Why do we need alternatives to institutional care? Are there any realistic alternatives to institutional care for persons suffering from such conditions as severe organic brain syndrome? Is it valid to assume that institutions cannot provide good care? What can be done to make institutional care more appropriate and more acceptable? Can cost-accountable alternatives be developed or designed?

Objectives for Older Americans

In this chapter we have attempted to describe some of the general issues and problems relating to the care of the elderly in the United States. No such discussion would be complete without reference to the national policy on aging, as detailed in Title I of the Older Americans Act,[13] which sets forth the following objectives for older Americans:

1. An adequate income
2. The best possible physical and mental health
3. Suitable housing
4. Full restoration and rehabilitation services
5. Opportunity for employment without age discrimination
6. Retirement in health, honor, and dignity
7. Pursuit of meaningful activity
8. Efficient community services when needed
9. Immediate benefit from proven research knowledge
10. Freedom, independence, and the free exercise of individual initiative

The achievement of these objectives, signed into law by

President Lyndon Johnson on July 14, 1965, could accomplish much in the way of solving problems of the aged in America. When and how will we achieve these objectives?

The nursing profession can make its specific contribution through the delivery of high-quality nursing and health services designed to promote individual health. These services should include understanding of the aging process, restorative care, health maintenance, and preventive care. To perform these services, nurses need to be prepared with education that provides not only basic competence in the care of the elderly, but also specialization in both community-based and high-quality institutional care, and training in conducting research directed toward the solution of nursing care problems.

3

The Study and Practice of Nursing the Aged

Historical Perspectives

Several of the basic concepts of gerontology were developed in the 1930s, according to Birren and Clayton.[1] One concept is that the problems of aging are complex and are best studied in an interdisciplinary context. A second concept is that aging represents an interaction between biological predisposition and the environment. Two important factors contributed to the impetus for the study of aging. The focus in medicine was shifting from infectious diseases to chronic diseases, which require consideration of the physiology of aging; and it was evident that the social and health problems of the increasing older population required attention. Around 1940, gerontology began to receive recognition as an important field of study.

Davis[2] dates the development of geriatric nursing as beginning about 1935, with the enactment of the Social Security Act. Because this Act made public assistance funds available to the needy aged who did not live in institutions, it became feasible for retired and widowed nurses and others to convert their homes to boarding homes. These boarding-house proprietors became the first geriatric practitioners and the first nursing home nurses.[3] It was not until after World War II that minimal standards were established for nursing home care and licensure of homes became a practice.

Thus, it is understandable that gerontic nursing as a specialty is not as far advanced as other specialty areas in nursing. State Boards do not require knowledge of it for licensure of registered nurses. But the continually increasing proportion of the population in the older age groups, together with their demand and needs for health services, have pushed gerontic nursing to the forefront of nursing. The needs for gerontic nurses, gerontic clinical specialists, geriatric practitioners for ambulatory care, teachers, researchers, and administrators in the field are unfulfilled. We are only beginning to appreciate the need for health specialists in adult health and aging as costs of medical care have escalated to a point where all individuals must be prepared to assume ever greater responsibilities for their own health care. Thus a new challenge exists for the promotion of health of the adult and aging proportions of the population.

It was not until 1962, when the ANA recommended the formation of special interest groups, that a group of geriatric nurses was formally organized. In 1966, the ANA established five divisions on nursing practice, one of which was the Division of Geriatric Nursing Practice.

In the June, 1968, editorial of *Nursing Outlook*,[4] it was noted that membership of the original special interest group (geriatrics) had grown from 70 nurses to 21,563. The editorial stated that in the future both nursing education and nursing research in geriatrics would have to concern themselves with:

1. Skill in the care of the elderly who have medical problems
2. The welfare of the aged within the family structure
3. Examination or assessment and acceptance of the limitations that occur in the aging process
4. The needs and morale of all personnel who work with the aged
5. Methods to alleviate the many social, physical, and emotional problems that affect or afflict the aged
6. The cultivation of less judgmental attitudes toward the aged

7. Good interpersonal relations skills for those who work with the elderly

In addition to the above concerns, nuring should now place considerably more emphasis on the promotion and maintenance of health in the aged, as well as on the achievement of human potential at advanced ages.

The currently prevailing definition of geriatric nursing in the United States was provided in 1970 by the ANA Committee on Standards for Geriatric Nursing Practice:

> Geriatric nursing is concerned with the assessment of nursing needs of older people, planning and implementing nursing care to meet these needs, and evaluating the effectiveness of such care to achieve and maintain a level of wellness consistent with the limitations imposed by the aging process.
>
> In the practice of geriatric nursing, the nurse adapts processes common to all nursing to the unique needs of older persons. These include: using problem-solving methods; working with families, co-workers, and community agencies; using knowledge and theories from nursing and basic applied sciences; extending knowledge through research and studies; and sharing knowledge through teaching and other communication media.
>
> In addition to these commonalities, there are primary factors which make the nursing of older persons different. Among these factors are the chronological age and the effect of the aging process; the multiplicity of the older person's losses, social, economic, psychologic, and biologic; the frequently atypical response of the aged to disease, coupled with the different forms disease entities may assume in the aged person; the accumulative disabling effect of multiple chronic illnesses and/or degenerative processes; and cultural values associated with aging and social attitudes toward the aged.[5]

In England, Doreen Norton (1965) provided a somewhat different concept of geriatric nursing.[6] She defined geriatrics as the positive approach to the preservation and restoration of human ability in old age. Then, for teaching purposes, she divided geriatric care into two parts: the physical management of the patient, including understanding of attitudes and behavior of old age, and the application of an intimate knowledge of the social aspects and problems of old people in the community. She described geriatric nursing practice as providing care for two categories of elderly sick: the rehabilitation category, consisting of patients who can regain the ability for basic self-care; and the irremediable category (geriatric long-stay or chronic), consisting of patients who are beyond medical reclaim and will need some degree of nursing care for the remainder of their lives. Norton emphasized the opportunities for nurses to learn the basic principles of nursing care in geriatric facilities.

Both of the definitions of care of the elderly presented above emphasize the need for careful assessment; the use of processes common to the nursing care of all groups; and the need for knowledge of the aging process, of the environments in which old people live, and of social support systems. Both also emphasize nursing attitudes and behavior. The description of the ANA Committee on Standards emphasizes the need for using theories and research findings and extending knowledge through research and publications. Norton's definition emphasizes that many of the older people needing and receiving nursing care are terminally ill and will need care that brings comfort, happiness, and peace of mind, since rehabilitation is not possible. This fact is only beginning to be grasped by those in geriatric practice in America.

A Definition of Gerontic Nursing

In 1976 the division of the ANA that is concerned with care of the aged was retitled *Division on Gerontological Nursing Practice,* and the standards for nursing practice were reformulated. Thus, it would seem that part of the evolutionary process of nursing the aged is finding the right name for it.

The term *geriatric* is derived from the Greek *geron* meaning "old man" and *iatros* meaning "healer" or "physician." Hence, *geriatrics* refers to a branch of medicine that deals with diseases of old people. Many in the profession objected to the term *geriatric nursing* because it seemed to mean nursing the aged who are ill. Hence the substitution of the term *gerontological nursing.*

The Study and Practice of Nursing the Aged

Some nurses object to this term because the suffix *ology* denotes "the scientific study" of some phenomenon—in the case of gerontology, the scientific study of old age. Some have even turned in desperation to the compound term *geriatric/gerontological nursing*. The present authors propose that, while there may someday be a nursing gerontology, just as there is now a social gerontology and a medical gerontology, the term is inappropriate to designate the *practice* of nursing the aged. We propose that the terminology dilemma be solved by simply getting rid of the offending suffixes *iatric* and *ology* and using the suffix *ic*, thus deriving the adjective *gerontic*, meaning "of or pertaining to old age." Hence, *gerontic nursing* means the nursing of the aged.

But a name is not a definition. The next task, then, is to define gerontic nursing. Gerontic nursing is proposed to be a health service that incorporates generic nursing methods and specialized knowledge about the aged to establish conditions within the client and/or within the environment that will:

1. Increase health-conducive behaviors in the aged
2. Minimize and compensate for health-prejudicial losses and impairments of aging
3. Provide comfort and sustenance through the distressing and debilitating events of aging including dying and death
4. Facilitate the diagnosis, palliation, and treatment of disease(s) in the aged

This definition attempts to specify the critical attributes of the concept gerontic nursing: *What* is it? Gerontic nursing is a health service for the aged. What are its aims? Its aims are to safeguard and increase health to the extent possible, and to provide comfort and care to the extent necessary. The health-directedness of the aims of gerontic nursing is one feature that distinguishes it from other helping professions. What are the means for accomplishing the aims? Gerontic nursing effects its aims through the health-relevant conditions that it can establish in the client and/or the environment. Conditions within the client include the cognitive and affective as well as the physical. Conditions within the environment include social as well as physical components.

What distinguishes gerontic nursing from nursing practice in other areas? The distinguishing feature is thought to be the acquisition by nurses of a body of knowledge about the health/aging/illness interactions in the aged and the utilization of that knowledge in making judgments, formulating realistic aims, specifying conditions, and choosing nursing methods appropriate for aged clients.

One implication of this view of gerontic nursing is that age is the important determinant of the nursing needs of clients and of the capabilities required of nurses in meeting those needs. To avoid misinterpretation (or accusations of "agism") it is necessary to qualify this statement. Most of us would agree that it is not chronological age per se that is important in gerontic nursing, but rather, some correlates of age. At present, age simply serves as an available index of these other variables that seem to be important in health and illness. If care is taken to avoid the error of assuming that the correlation between chronological age and the important variables is perfect, then age can serve as a useful index to client characteristics until a better one can be found. Age is at least a starting point for making the teaching of nursing manageable and, more fundamentally, for determining whether nursing the aging is something that can be taught.

To illustrate more concretely the meaning and the implications of this definition, let us consider a few examples. The definition suggests that the first event following the initiation of a health care service is the search for some evidence of disease, distress, health decrement, or health deficit. In addition to the observation skills required for collecting evidence about any client, particular knowledge about aging and the health/aging/illness interaction is necessary if nurses are to know what evidence to look for. Only someone with a notion of what constitutes health in old age can recognize when there is a decrement or deficit. Knowledge is also necessary if nurses are to appropriately interpret and use the evidence they collect. A simple example can illustrate this point. Temperature-regulating mechanisms are less reliable in the elderly, consequently, in an infection, fever may appear late, may not reach very high levels, or may not appear at all. In fact, a *decrease* in body temperature often constitutes important evidence in the aged. Thus, interpretation of "temperature evidence" by nurses whose knowledge of temperature responses is confined to those typical of children or young adults, might result in serious error. Once evidence has been used to make some judgments about whether a client is suffering from some deficit, decrement, distress, or disease, the next task is to determine achievable nursing aims. Here again, accurate knowledge is crucial. For example, negative stereotypical views of the aged seem likely to interfere with judgments agout nursing aims because they lead to underestimation of patients' abilities. Aims may be restricted simply to sustenance or palliation when they should be directed toward compensation or restoration. Such incorrect judgments might make the difference between institutionalizing a client and maintaining him in the community. On the other hand, aims that are unrealistically high can also be detrimental. For instance, nurses aware of the benefits of activity, but with expectations based on physical reserve capacities of adolescents or young adults, may fail to help their aged clients, not because they neglect them but because they exhaust them! Here again, specific knowledge and the ability to relate it to the care of aged clients are important.

Thus, it is essential to determine what conditions within the client and/or within the environment must be established (or modified) in order to achieve the aims of health, compensation, sustenance, and so on. Safe and effective nursing requires that nurses learn to organize these conditions into three categories:

1. Conditions that can be established through nursing expertise alone
2. Conditions that can be established in collaboration with other health care workers
3. Conditions that are outside the range of nursing expertise and require referral to other resources

The ability to identify and establish conditions that are appropriate to the achievement of the nursing aims requires sophisticated capabilities, including skill in appropriate nursing methods. Consider again the example of nurses whose knowledge is limited to children or young adults. When such a nurse is confronted with an aged client who pays absolutely no attention to what the nurse says, is it realistic to expect the nurse to *intuitively* relate this evidence to a possible hearing deficit? Perhaps, but how likely is the nurse to quickly figure out a simple set of actions that might effect compensation: modifying oral communication by speaking more slowly and lowering the pitch of her voice? Or, another example—unless nurses are instructed about the nature of visual changes in the aged and about how this knowledge can be used in modifying the environment, it seems unlikely that they will know that appropriate color conditions may help compensate for visual decrements.

This kind of interaction, of course, encompasses a wider concept of nursing service than simple, direct nurse-client contact or physically-oriented actions. For example, the patient may give evidence of psychological distress associated with some event such as loss of a spouse. The nurse then seeks to establish a comforting and sustaining environmental condition. She can involve family members and/or use herself to provide a condition of appropriate comforting and sustaining social interaction.

A final implication of our definition of gerontic nursing is that once nurses have found the evidence related to health status and attempted to establish appropriate conditions to achieve nursing aims, they have not arrived at the *end* of a nursing process. Rather, they have come full circle and are back once more at the beginning. And back at the beginning the task is to collect evidence of deficits, decrement, distress, or disease. If any such evidence is again found, it is the signal to move to the next step and look once more for appropriate nursing aims. In a cyclic concept of nursing, nursing never *appropriately* ends until the client is either in perfect health (has no health deficit) or is dead. It may, of course, end *inappropriately* at any phase within the cycle because of error, technical constraints, or other human limitations.

The cyclic concept holds true even at the simple levels used here for illustration, for example, the aged client who did not respond to verbal input. This was posed as evidence of a *decrement* in hearing. The nursing aim of compensating for the loss was selected and the decision made to establish in the environment an auditory condition to compensate for the decrement (lowering the pitch of the voice and decreasing the rate of speech communication). This brings the nurse not to the end of any process, but back at the beginning of the cycle looking again for evidence. What is the evidence this second time around? If it is essentially the same as before, then something went wrong in the cycle. The evidence may have been interpreted incorrectly—perhaps inattention was *not* related to a hearing decrement. The nursing aim of compensation may have been unachieveable. Perhaps instead the nurse should have decided the best aim would be to facilitate diagnosis of disease, and call a physician. Finally, perhaps the nurse only thought she had established the desired condition. Maybe she thought she spoke lower and slower, but she only spoke louder. This simple example illustrates the complexity of nursing—the information, the judgments, and the skills that are required.

The basic premise of the views presented here is that nursing care of the aged constitutes a distinct nursing practice area that is distinguishable from other nursing practice areas. Its uniqueness rests mainly in its knowledge component and in nursing method adaptations designed to meet the special needs of the aged.

Nursing Gerontology Defined

Gerontology is defined as the study of the aging processes in man and animals which, for practical purposes, is further divided into biological, psychological, and social aging. Havighurst has stated that, as an applied science, gerontology utilizes the knowledge of aging to make life longer and more satisfying, but as a pure science, it seeks knowledge about the aging process in humans and animals, as individuals and in population groups. According to Havighurst, the field of applied gerontology consists of medical and social divisions, each consisting of three aspects. *"Medical gerontology* includes: (1) treatment of the elderly patient, (2) prevention of disease and disability in the elderly, and (3) preservation of vigor in the elderly. *Social gerontology* considers: (1) financial support of the elderly, (2) housing and living arrangements of the elderly, and (3) ego support of the elderly."[7] It is here proposed that there is also a third applied field—nursing gerontology.

Nursing gerontology is defined as the scientific study of the nursing care of the elderly. It is characterized as an applied science since its aim is to use knowledge of the aging process to design nursing care and services that best provide for the health, longevity, and independence or highest level of functioning possible in the aging and aged. The concept of nursing gerontology is derived from consideration of the definition of gerontology, as well as definitions of geriatrics, geriatric nursing, and nursing research.

Geriatric Nursing Defined

Geriatrics is the term applied to the medical treatment of disease in the elderly. The ANA definition of geriatric nursing presented earlier in this chapter[8] stresses the provision of care that is consistent with the limitations imposed by the aging process. On the other hand, Norton[9] defines geriatrics as the positive approach to the preservation and the restoration of human ability in old age, as was discussed earlier.

But what is missing in both of these definitions of geriatric nursing is the health promotional aspect, wherein nurses assist the aging and aged to understand the aging process, to separate the effects of aging from disease, and to control the aging process through use of hygenic practices and life styles that promote health, vigor, and attractiveness into old age, and prevent some of the pathological conditions that accompany aging when the principles of healthful living are disregarded.

To further explicate the concept of nursing gerontology, it is necessary to speak briefly about research and, more specifically, nursing research. Nursing gerontology would fit what Abdellah and Levine[10] defined as applied research—that designed to obtain facts and/or identify relationships among facts that are intended to be used in a naturalistic situation. Its purposes are problem solving, decision making, or developing or evaluating programs, procedures, processes, or products. Nursing gerontology fits this definition of applied nursing research because of its aims of improving nursing care and services, institutional and home care, and promoting health maintenance, rehabilitation, and supportive services for the elderly. Particular attention is given to the nursing process, organization of services, and the training of nursing personnel in the delivery of health services to the aging population.

Interaction of Research and Practice

Although for expository purposes, the fields of gerontic nursing and nursing gerontology have been defined and treated separately, and their distinctive characteristics elaborated, this is not to imply that they are not interacting components of a functional whole—nursing. Nursing care of the aged is the concern of both the nurse gerontologist and the gerontic nurse. The former is concerned with the scientific *study* of nursing the aged, the latter with the *practice* of nursing the aged. Knowledge about aging is valued by both researcher and practitioner. The goal of the one is expansion of knowledge to benefit the aged; the goal of the other is application of knowledge to benefit the aged.

Put another way, common nursing knowledge about health and illness and common nursing methods necessary to provide care of elderly persons are derived from nursing in general. Additional specific knowledge about the aging person is derived from the science of gerontology. The aging person is undergoing both health-illness and aging processes, i.e., he is experiencing a health/aging/illness interaction. Knowledge of this interaction and modifications of nursing care required on the basis of this interaction constitute the special aspects of gerontic nursing. The nursing gerontologist studies this phenomenon; the practicing gerontic nurse applies knowledge and methods derived from the study.

Figure 3-1 depicts a derivation of nursing gerontology and gerontic nursing from this viewpoint, and shows graphically the contributions of each of the relevant fields of endeavor to nursing care of the aged. Figure 3-2 depicts the interactive nature of the component disciplines by showing both their unique and shared domains of concern. The overriding concern of all is the aged population.

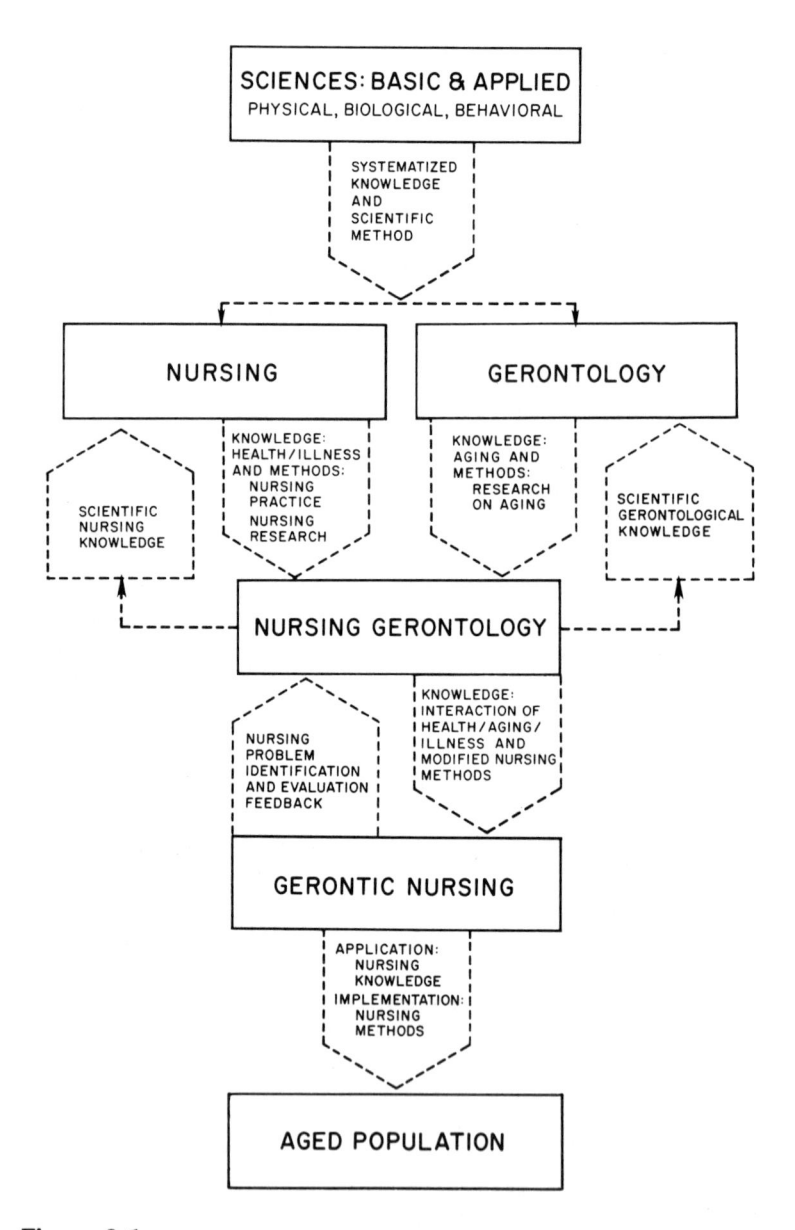

Figure 3-1.
The Derivation of Nursing Gerontology and Gerontic Nursing

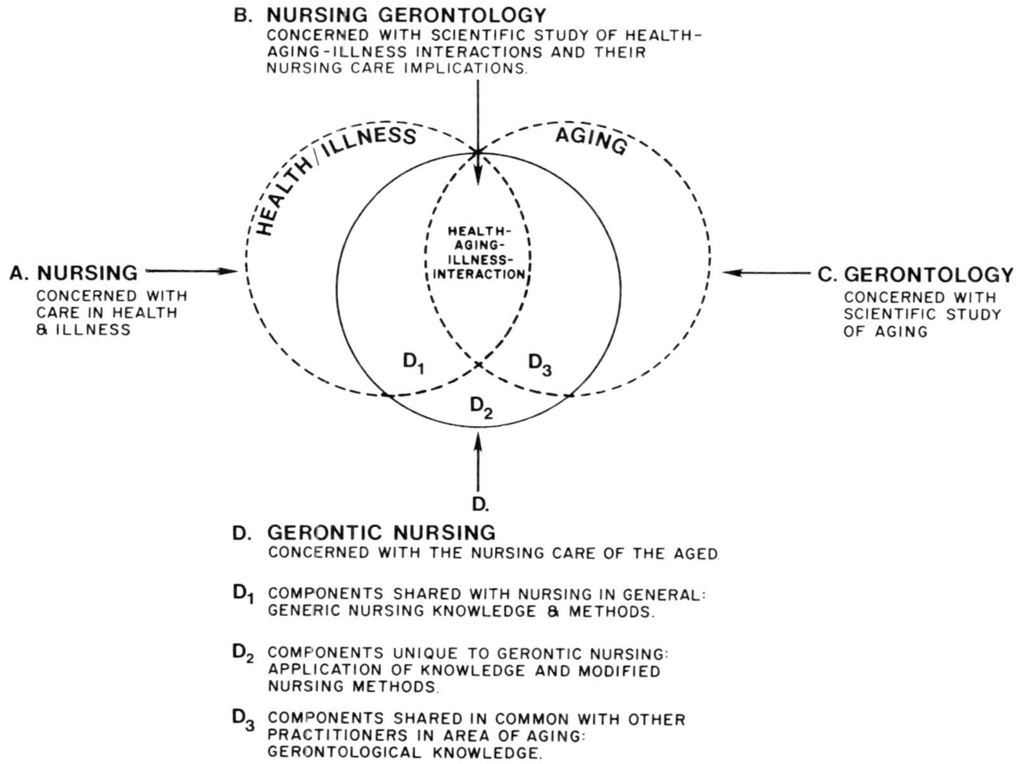

B. NURSING GERONTOLOGY
CONCERNED WITH SCIENTIFIC STUDY OF HEALTH-AGING-ILLNESS INTERACTIONS AND THEIR NURSING CARE IMPLICATIONS.

C. GERONTOLOGY
CONCERNED WITH SCIENTIFIC STUDY OF AGING

A. NURSING
CONCERNED WITH CARE IN HEALTH & ILLNESS

D. GERONTIC NURSING
CONCERNED WITH THE NURSING CARE OF THE AGED

D_1 COMPONENTS SHARED WITH NURSING IN GENERAL: GENERIC NURSING KNOWLEDGE & METHODS.

D_2 COMPONENTS UNIQUE TO GERONTIC NURSING: APPLICATION OF KNOWLEDGE AND MODIFIED NURSING METHODS.

D_3 COMPONENTS SHARED IN COMMON WITH OTHER PRACTITIONERS IN AREA OF AGING: GERONTOLOGICAL KNOWLEDGE.

Figure 3-2. The Domains of Concern in Nursing and Aging: Unique and Overlapping Components

4
Preparing the Nurse's Aide for Gerontic Nursing*

The Function of the Nurse's Aide

Nurses' aides are employed and trained "to perform tasks that involve specified services for patients as delegated by the professional nurse and performed under the direction of professional nurses or licensed practical nurses."[1]

In their 1962 statement on Training for Health Occupations,[2] the steering committee for the National League for Nursing's (NLN) Department of Practical Nursing Programs emphasized the fact that nurses' aides are not nurses, and discouraged the establishment of short-term preservice programs for a variety of nursing assistants. While they recognized a shortage of nurses, they defined this as a shortage of nurses for administrative, supervisory, and teaching positions which were unfilled, or filled by persons with less than the desirable level of educational preparation. This shortage could not be remedied by the training of nurses' assistants.

A 1962 editorial in *Nursing Outlook*[3] stated that employers should be clear about what the nurse's aide should do, as well as about how the aide should be trained. The nurse's aide should

*The authors acknowledge the assistance of Joanne Ryan in the preparation of this chapter.

not be assigned to a patient but to a task. Licensing of the aide was not then, and is not now, supported by the ANA or the NLN, nor do the aide's activities constitute the practice of nursing. One of the major problems in nursing is the reversal of the duties of the nurse's aide and the nurse; the aide no longer functions as an assistant to the licensed nurse but carries out the role of the licensed nurse, who has now often become the aide's assistant. Too frequently, the nurse functions only in a supervisory or assisting role and is no longer involved in direct patient care, although she is still legally and ethically responsible for the patient's care. Thus, the nurse has, in a sense, delegated her responsibilities to the aide, particularly in nursing homes, but to some extent in hospitals, too.

The present ambiguous state of nursing as a profession can be traced back to the delegation of nursing functions to other health workers and of assistive functions (assistant to the physician and assistant to the auxiliary workers) to nurses. One recent counter-trend is the implementation of the concept of primary nursing, which is nothing more than the involvement of the nurse in direct patient care with assistance from auxiliary personnel. This is what was intended when auxiliary personnel were first introduced into nursing services.

Sister Marilyn Schwab[4] has emphasized the fact that effective primary care cannot be given by nurses' aides. Her thesis is that nursing care is effective only when it is planned, based on sound data about the patient and sound theory about intervention, and evaluated continuously. Nurses have an obligation to resume responsibility for the direct patient care of the aged. From this perspective, we do not believe that extensive preservice training programs for aides should be supplied. We do not support the practice of providing mini-schools of nursing for aides. We do support the use of auxiliary nursing personnel in well-organized nursing services, where policies and procedures are written and followed, where adequate personnel policies are in effect, where orientation and in-service programs are available, and where licensed nurses provide direct care. These conditions are made explicit in the following curriculum design for the training of nurses' aides to function as assistants to nurses.

Curriculum Design for On-the-job Training for the Nurse's Aide

Assumption: We believe nurses' aides should work under the direct supervision of registered nurses and/or licensed practical nurses. Therefore:

1. An orientation to agency philosophy, policies, procedures, and environment is required for all nursing personnel
2. An apprentice relationship with a licensed nurse should be established for each nurse's aide
3. Nurses may need assistance in understanding their legal and ethical responsibilities for aides who assist them in providing nursing care and in understanding their responsibilities to teach, guide, and advise the aide
4. In-service programs that provide for the solution of current conflicts and problems between nurses' aides, patients, or licensed nurses are essential for the optimal operation of nursing services
5. An understanding of roles, functions, and responsibilities of nursing personnel and all other persons within the institution or home environment is needed for all personnel
6. An understanding of the basic ethical and legal aspects of providing nursing service to consumers is needed for all nursing personnel
7. An understanding of the purposes of supervision and of inservice education programs in needed by all nursing personnel

Assumption: We believe the licensed nurse must assign tasks to be performed as necessary by the nurse's aide to supplement self-care activities for the aged in institutions and home care programs. Thus, the nurse's aide must have:

1. Sufficient knowledge to appreciate the importance of safe physical care of the aged within the framework of preservation and restoration of function in a safe environment

2. Basic knowledge and skill in selected aspects of safe physical care
3. A basic knowledge of physiological and psychosocial aspects of aging that have direct relevance to assigned tasks
4. Basic knowledge and work skills necessary to maintain a safe and hygienic environment
5. Basic knowledge and skills for carrying out selected measures that contribute to preservation and restoration of functions

Assumption: Since nurses' aides will spend considerable time with patients, they should be prepared to establish a relationship supportive to the aged. Training should include acquiring skill in the following aspects of communication:

1. Establishing friendships
2. Using touch and space
3. Giving directions while assisting patients
4. Speaking to deaf patients
5. Speaking to aphasic patients
6. Listening
7. Perceiving nonverbal forms of communication
8. Persuading
9. Communicating to nurses and other workers
10. Correctly interpreting directions from nurses and those components of nursing care plans directly related to assigned tasks.
11. Recording data

Basic knowledge and skills for performing a helping role in the application of psychosocial techniques useful in nursing should be taught, including those involving remotivation, reality orientation, and reinforcement techniques. Additional knowledge and skills may be appropriately taught to especially capable aides, but those aides with the required ability and motivation may be guided into formal programs for the preparation of licensed nurses.

Expected Competencies for the Nurse's Aide in Gerontic Nursing

The nurse's aide in gerontic nursing should be able to demonstrate:

1. Knowledge of the philosophy, policies, and procedures of the employing agency
2. Knowledge of responsibilities in assisting licensed nurses, the family, or the client in providing nursing care
3. Psychomotor skills for carrying out selected measures designed to preserve function
4. Skills for maintaining a safe environment
5. Awareness of common psychosocial problems of aging
6. Observation skills sufficient to recognize obvious changes in physical and psychosocial functioning
7. Competence in communication skills
8. Knowledge of an aide's ethical and legal responsibilities to patients/clients, families, professional staff, and agency

Developing an On-the-job Training Program

Description

The nurse's aide in gerontic nursing, whose background preparation should include, at minimum, an eighth-grade education, should be trained to function as an assistant to the licensed nurse in the care of aged individuals with physiological and psychosocial needs. General health problems of the aged will be considered, and correlated laboratory practice and clinical experience will be provided. It is suggested the program run four weeks of intensive training for new personnel, and five lectures and five laboratory hours, along with supervised work experiences each week for 12 weeks, for those presently employed.

Objectives

The program should train the aide to:
1. Know function and responsibility as member of health team
2. Know physiological and psychosocial aspects of aging relevant to the aide's level of functioning
3. Give selected aspects of care skillfully and safely to aged persons under direction of licensed staff nurses
4. Communicate effectively with aged persons and staff according to the situation

Course Content

The Training Program Outline and unit modules shown in Table 4-1 are suggested for use in on-the-job training programs for preparing nurses' aides to work in the field of gerontic nursing. The learning activities suggested for this program include lectures, tours, discussion, slide demonstration, practice, clinical observation, films, and video tape, to be selected as appropriate for the topic of the learning activity.

Table 4-1.
Training Program Outline for the Nurse's Aide in Gerontic Nursing

Unit 1. Orientation to Working Environments	
Objectives	*Content*
At the completion of this unit, the student will be able to:	1. Role of the aide
1. Specify major facilities of institutions (nursing homes, rehabilitation centers, hospitals)	2. General philosophy of the care of the aged
2. Know general layout and equipment of an institutional unit (ward, floor, etc.)	3. Facilities for nutrition
	4. Facilities for environmental sanitation
3. Identify basic equipment in a patient unit	5. Facilities for safety (including fire regulations)
4. Identify selected personnel, administrative structure, and duties	6. Facilities for personal activities of daily living
	7. Facilities for medical care (therapy, pharmacy)
5. Identify minimal facilities required for the elderly in the home	8. Administrative structures
	9. Team responsibilities
	10. Community resources

Preparing the Nurse's Aide

Table 4-1. *(continued)*
6. List common community resources
7. Understand the patient is a guest in an institution
8. Understand that a health worker in the home is a guest
9. State general philosophy of the care of the aging

Unit 2. Maintaining a Safe, Clean, Orderly Environment	
Objectives	*Content*
At the completion of this unit the student will be able to:	1. Safety in an institution
1. Identify safety measures	a. for patients
2. Identify unsafe equipment obstacles	b. for personnel
3. Identify safety habits of patients and personnel	c. for visitors
4. Practice correct body mechanics	2. Safety in the home
	a. for elderly
	b. for family
	c. for health worker
	3. Body mechanics
	a. correct body posture and alignment
	b. moving and stooping
	c. lifting

Unit 3. Physiological and Psychosocial Aspects of Aging	
Objectives	*Content*
At the completion of this unit the student will be expected to:	1. Physical signs of aging, as shown by changes in:
1. Identify outward physical signs of aging	a. the integument
2. Know general physiological aspects of aging in patients with:	b. muscles and posture
a. cardiovascular disorders	c. gait and movements
b. pulmonary-renal disorders	d. dress and habits
c. gastrointestinal disorders	2. Physiological aspects of aging, as they affect the:
d. integumentary disorders	a. cardiovascular system
e. sensory organ disorders	b. pulmonary system
f. musculoskeletal disorders	c. renal system
3. Know physiological effects of rest	d. gastrointestinal system
4. Know general psychosocial aspects of aging	e. sensory system
	f. integumentary system
	3. Psychosocial aspects of aging, as they affect the patients':
	a. family and friends
	b. productivity
	c. financial status
	d. independence
	e. psychological reactions
	f. sociological implications
	g. environment

Table 4-1. (*continued*)

Unit 4. Activities of Daily Living

Objectives

At the completion of this unit, the student will be able to:
1. Deduct the rationale for promoting activities of daily living (ADL) from preceding units
2. Give a complete and partial bed bath, a tub bath, skin inspection, and skin care
3. Give oral hygiene and denture care
4. Give hair and nail care
5. Position patients in normal body alignment
6. Give passive range of motion (PROM) and teach active range of motion exercises
7. Assist a person to feed himself or feed a person
8. Assist a person in dressing
9. Assist a person in safe transfer
10. Assist a person in active exercises, walking
11. Encourage a person to participate, set goals, and achieve satisfaction in social activities

Content

1. Review rationale for activity
2. Personal hygiene
    a. bathing
    b. hair
    c. nails
    d. dentures
3. Nutrition
    a. feeding
    b. socialization while eating
    c. fluids
4. Muscular activities
    a. passive ROM
    b. active ROM
    c. active resistive ROM
5. Rest
    a. bed and sleep
    b. positioning
    c. sitting in alignment and safety
6. Dressing activities
7. Socialization
    a. group participation
    b. one-to-one interpersonal interaction
    c. goals
    d. pleasure in achievement

Unit 5. Observational Skills

Objectives

At the completion of this unit, the student will be able to:
1. Take and record oral, rectal, and skin temperatures
2. Care for thermometers
3. Take and record pulse and respirations
4. Observe, record, and report bowel habits
5. Observe, measure, and record fluid intake and output
6. Observe and record dietary habits and intake
7. Observe and report patients' general physical condition, as learned in Unit 4
8. Observe and report patients' social and psychological state and interactions, as learned in Unit 4

Content

1. Vital signs
    a. temperature
    b. pulse
    c. respiration
    d. care of equipment
    e. recording and reporting
2. Nutrition and eating habits
    a. importance
    b. observation
    c. reporting
3. Fluid balance
    a. importance
    b. intake
    c. output
4. Bowel habits
5. Review physical, physiological and psychosocial state
    a. mood changes
    b. activities
    c. behavioral and physical changes

Table 4-1. (continued)

Unit 6. Communication Skills

Objectives	Content

At the completion of this unit, the student will be expected to:
1. Know that man is unique in having speech
2. Know that communication is an interactive process
3. Listen and give feedback as to acknowledgement, clarification, etc.
4. Recognize manipulative communication skills such as emotional appeal, authority, threat, hidden agendas
5. Give exact factual data without value judgments or connotative expressions
6. Be alert to nonverbal cues and implications
7. Be honest in communication
8. Be reciprocal in communication
9. Acknowledge all communication
	1. Factors that influence communication
	2. Communication as a process
	3. Feedback
	  a. verbal
	  b. nonverbal
	4. Dishonest communication
	  a. control
	  b. threat
	  c. fear
	  d. hidden agendas
	5. Factual reports
	6. Friendship skills
	  a. acknowledgement of another person
	  b. prevention of attack and insult
	  c. reciprocity
	  d. acknowledgement of communication
	  e. confidentiality of communication

Unit 7. Rehabilitative Measures

Objectives	Content

At the completion of this unit, the student will be able to:
1. State principles of rehabilitation
2. Describe general causes of brain damage
3. Differentiate right from left stroke signs and symptoms
4. Position stroke patients in lying, sitting, and standing situations
5. Help stroke patients relearn ADL
6. Perform activities with stroke patients
7. Communicate with stroke patients
8. Assist arthritic patients in ADL
9. Assist amputee patients in ADL
10. Appreciate psychosocial problems of patients with physical disabilities other than aging
11. Assist patients with reality orientation
	1. Principles of rehabilitation
	  a. preservation of function
	  b. restoration of function
	2. Stroke
	  a. signs and symptoms
	  b. preservation of function
	  c. utilization of abilities
	  d. problems in communication
	  e. communication measures
	3. Arthritis
	  a. osteoarthritis and rheumatoid arthritis
	  b. suspected etiologies
	  c. signs and symptoms
	  d. measures for preservation of function
	  e. appreciation of pain
	  f. measures for maintenance of function
	4. Amputees
	  a. reasons for amputation
	  b. preservation of function

Table 4-1. (continued)

      c. utilization of abilities
5. Psychological impact of disability
    a. denial
    b. mourning
    c. hostility
    d. withdrawal
    e. regression
    f. acceptance
6. The confused patient
7. Possible sociological implications

Unit 8. Bowel and Bladder Training

Objectives	Content

At the completion of this unit, the student will be able to:
1. State rationale for bowel and bladder training and methods
2. Assist in bowel and bladder training
3. Observe and report results of training
	1. Review rationale for training from Unit 4
	2. Anatomy and physiology of colon
	3. Relationship of food and fluids to colonic function
	4. Methods
	  a. diet (bulk-roughage)
	  b. fluids
	  c. regularity
	  d. abdominal and pelvic muscles
	  e. positioning
	  f. psychological factors
	  g. suppositories
	    1. types
	    2. action
	    3. method of insertion
	  h. enemas
	    1. types
	    2. action
	    3. method of irrigation
	  i. bladder training
	    1. fluids
	    2. timing
	    3. impulses
	    4. psychological factors
	    5. care of catheters
	    6. anatomical structure
	    7. asepsis
	    8. skin care
	  j. exercise

Table 4-1. (continued)

Unit 9. Adaptive Equipment

Objectives	Content

At the completion of this unit, the student will be able to:
1. State general purpose of adaptive equipment
2. Use specific adaptive equipment safely for ADL
  a. Hoyer lifts
  b. bath lifts
  c. wheelchairs
  d. transfer belts
  e. side rails
  f. eating equipment
  g. bathroom safety equipment
  h. walkers, canes
  i. braces and splints
  j. slings
  k. Velcro
  l. crutches
  m. hearing aids
  n. eyeglasses
	1. Adaptive devices to assist functional abilities
	2. Safety devices
	3. Specific devices
	  a. Hoyer lifts
	  b. bath lifts
	  c. wheelchairs
	  d. transfer belts
	  e. side rails
	  f. eating equipment
	  g. bathroom safety equipment
	  h. walkers, canes
	  i. braces and splints
	  j. slings
	  k. Velcro
	  l. crutches
	  m. hearing aids
	  n. eyeglasses

Unit 10. Caring for a Person with Diabetes

Objectives	Content

At the completion of this unit, the student will be able to:
1. Describe general signs and symptoms of diabetes mellitus
2. Identify general reasons for urinalysis, blood tests, diets, exercise, medication, from general knowledge of pathology
3. Assist patients with nutrition, activities, and acceptance of living patterns
4. Observe and report signs, symptoms, habits
5. Test urine specimens
6. Observe and report food intake.
7. Recognize signs of coma and insulin shock.
	1. Diabetes mellitus
	  a. General signs and symptoms
	  b. Tests
	  c. Diet
	  d. Medication
	    1. insulin
	    2. oral hypoglycenic agents
	  e. emphasis on hygiene
	  f. importance of exercise
	  g. observation of signs and symptoms
	  h. urine testing
	  i. signs of coma and shock
	  j. importance of hygiene

Table 4-1. (*continued*)

Unit 11. Caring for a Person with Cardiovascular and/or Respiratory Problems	
Objectives	*Content*

At the completion of this unit, the student will be able to:
1. Know general function of heart as pump
2. Know importance of work and rest periods of heart
3. Know general pathology of myocardial infarction, cardiac decompensation
4. Know general measures for treatment
5. Know adjustment of ADL within patient's capacity and medical regime
	1. The heart as a pump
	   a. general anatomy
	   b. general function
	2. Signs and symptoms of heart problems
	3. Treatment
	4. ADL
	5. Precautions to be used in care of the patient receiving oxygen

Unit 12. Care of the Dying and Dead	
Objectives	*Content*

At the completion of this unit, the student will be able to:
1. Know physical signs and symptoms of death and dying
2. Know psychological adjustments to death
3. Identify family reactions to death
4. Care for the dying
5. Care for the dead
	1. Signs and symptoms of dying
	   a. physiological
	   b. psychological
	2. Care of the dying
	   a. physiological
	   b. psychological
	3. Care of the dead

5

Preparing the Licensed Practical Nurse for Gerontic Nursing

Given the NLN's statement of functions and qualifications of the licensed practical nurse (LPN),[1] one can assume that these nurses have the general or basic knowledge needed to provide care to all age groups. Gerontic nursing requires both general or basic knowledge and special knowledge of the aging process—gerontologic knowledge. Preparation of the licensed practical nurse for gerontic nursing may be accomplished by credit courses or continuing education.

Recent emphasis on career mobility makes the credit modality more attractive to those whose career goal is to become registered nurses. The authors recommend the baccalaureate degree, inasmuch as the associate degree program usually does not provide courses in gerontology or geriatric nursing. Courses in gerontology should be accessible within the baccalaureate program, and it is expected that courses in gerontic nursing will become more available, at least as electives.

Continuing education programs would provide the same training in gerontic nursing for licensed practical nurses as for registered nurses whose basic preparation did not include this content. Continuing education courses for licensed practical nurses would, therefore, include: the aging process; assessment; nursing intervention; psychosocial techniques; use of community resources; clinical problems; nursing process; and nursing team responsibilities and relationships.

To offer courses that will be given to both licensed practical nurses and registered nurses should foster the concept espoused by the NLN that the licensed practical nurse should be viewed by the registered nurse as a well-prepared coworker and should also help bring about a good team relationship and mutual respect. Further, such a system could contribute to cost-effectiveness in providing continuing education courses, and possibly lower the fees for such courses.

While the NLN suggests that continuing education courses dealing with direct patient care should provide clinical practice correlated with theory, this procedure has not been widely implemented. Perhaps a more feasible procedure would be to provide on-the-job consultation as a follow-up of continuing education classes and to encourage a team of two or more nurses to attend the same program. The nurses in the team could support each other in implementing changes on the job and strengthen the process by follow-up consultation. The additional content that would need to be provided for preparation in gerontic nursing would not necessarily involve the attainment of new motor skills but would be directed more toward understanding how the effects of aging interact to contribute to the present problems and how the nurses could make modifications in care to obtain desired results. For this reason, the combining of theory and practice in continuing education courses in gerontic nursing may be far less necessary than, for example, in courses in intensive care where the aim is to help the nurses develop new manual skills.

The premise of this chapter, then, is that licensed practical nurses are prepared in general or basic nursing to provide nursing care to the elderly. What they need in order to work effectively and therapeutically with the elderly is an understanding of the aging process, the interaction between this process and health, and the modifications that must be made in nursing activities to provide safe and effective care to the elderly.

Curriculum Design for In-service and Continuing Education for Practical Nurses

Assumption: The "practice of practical nursing" means the performance of selected nursing acts in the care of the ill, injured, or infirm under the direction of a licensed professional nurse, a licensed physician, or a licensed dentist that do not require the specialized skill, judgment, and knowledge required in professional nursing.[2]

The practical nurse is prepared to provide basic personal care to elderly clients in institutions and homes. The practical nurse can provide nursing services to clients as a member of a team of health professionals. The employing agency should sponsor planned programs of in-service education or continuing education that can provide the practical nurse with opportunities to obtain intensive preparation in specialized areas, in this case, gerontic nursing. Individuals who wish to change career goals should have the opportunity to do so. Licensed practical nurses who wish to become registered nurses should have the opportunity to enroll in formal educational programs designed for this purpose.

Assumption: The licensed practical nurse is prepared to carry out functions that are applicable to the care of the elderly, including providing for the emotional and physical comfort and safety of patients through:

1. Understanding human relationships between and among patients, families, and other health care personnel
2. Participating in the development, revision, and implementation of policies and procedures designed to ensure comfort and safety of patients and health-care personnel
3. Assisting the patient with activities of daily living and encouraging appropriate self-care.

4. Recognizing and understanding the effects of social and economic problems upon patients
5. Protecting patients from behavior that would damage their self-esteem or relationship with families, other patients, or other people
6. Recognizing and understanding cultural backgrounds and spiritual needs and respecting patients' religious beliefs
7. Considering the patients' needs for an attractive, comfortable, and safe environment

The practical nurse should be able to observe, record, and report to the appropriate persons about:

1. General and specific physical and mental conditions of patients, and signs and symptoms that may be indicative of change
2. Stresses in human relationships between patients, patients' families, visitors, and health care personnel.

The practical nurse should perform such specialized functions as:[3]

1. Administering prescribed medications and therapeutic treatments
2. Preparing and caring for patients receiving special treatments
3. Carrying out first aid, emergency, and disaster measures.

The practical nurse should be able to assist with rehabilitation of patients, according to the patient care plan, by:

1. Utilizing and applying the principles of prevention of deformities (e.g., the normal range of motion exercises, body mechanics, and body alignment)
2. Encouraging patients to help themselves within their capabilities
3. Being aware of the special aptitudes and interests of patients and encouraging their use
4. Utilizing community resources and facilities for continuing patient care.

The practical nurse who works with geriatric patients needs special post-basic preparation in:
1. The aging process
2. The nursing process
3. Nursing intervention
4. Psychosocial techniques
5. The use of community resources
6. Clinical problems
7. Nursing team relationships and responsibilities
8. Support systems

The important and substantial contribution of licensed practical nurses to the care of the aged should be recognized by nurses at all other levels of training.

Competencies for the Licensed Practical Nurse

At the completion of a beginning continuing (or in-service) education program in gerontic nursing, it is expected that the LPN will be able to demonstrate knowledge of:

1. The biological, sociological, and psychological aspects of the aging process
2. Dying and death as normal life events
3. Ways of promoting and maintaining health and a satisfying life through old age
4. Common problems arising from normal aging as well as disease
5. Common causes of illness and death among the aged
6. Nursing measures that are effective in illness and impairments of the aging, including responsibilities in drug therapy and rehabilitation
7. Special nursing methods, including maintenance of a therapeutic milieu and reality orientation
8. Effective approaches for establishing supportive interpersonal relationships
9. Community resources available for the aged.

Suggested Modules for Continuing Education Programs for Licensed Practical Nurses

The following unit modules (Table 5-1) are suggested for use in an in-service training program for preparing licensed practical nurses for gerontic nursing. Learning activities suggested for use with these modules include lectures, demonstration, discussions, textbook assignments, role playing, films and filmstrips, written reports, self-evaluation, and teacher-designed tests.

Table 5-1.
Unit Modules for Use in an In-service Training Program

Module 1. Aging as a Normal Process	
Objectives	*Content*

Identify major societal aspects of aging in the U.S.
Distinguish common myths and stereotypes from realities of aging
	Aging in our society:
	  Overview (demography)
	  Social concern and legislation
	  Attitudes and stereotypes

Recognize aging, dying, and death as part of normal life process
Recognize common biological, psychological and sociological concomitants of aging
	Aging as normal development:
	  Developmental tasks of the aged
	  Psychological aspects of aging

Describe ways of improving psychosocial need fulfillment
Specify ways of accommodating to the physical changes common to aging
Identify the needs common to the dying
Specify ways a nurse may meet the dying person's needs
	Social aspects of aging:
	  Meeting psychosocial needs
	  Physical changes of aging
	  Accommodating to physical changes
	  Dying and death

Module 2. Nursing to Promote Health and Quality of Life for the Aged	
Objectives	*Content*

List common causes of accidents among the aged
Describe measures for preventing common accidents
Recognize safety hazards in an environmental setting
Recognize the importance of physical care and grooming
	Personal care and safety:
	  Prevention of injury
	  Physical care and grooming
	  Activities of daily living
	  Nutrition

Preparing the Licensed Practical Nurse

Table 5-1. *(continued)*

Identify ways of assisting and involving the aged in their activities of daily living Relate characteristics of aging to common nutritional problems Describe approaches to solving common nutrition problems in the aged	

Identify basic human "life satisfaction" needs
Name major types of community resources for the aged.
	The aged: their continuing needs and resources:
	  Appropriate housing
	  Economic security
	  Useful activity
	  Recreation
	  Accessible health care
	  Sexual expression

Module 3. Special Skills in Gerontic Nursing

Objectives	*Content*

Define assessment as collecting and evaluating information about a client
Recognize the purpose of assessment is to identify the needs and problems of clients and the kind of care that will be effective
Demonstrate ability to collect appropriate assessment data systematically
Identify factors important in assessing the physical environment of the aged
Identify categories of physical capabilities important in assessment
Identify focuses for assessing psychosocial function
Specify characteristics of measurable objectives
Formulate measurable objectives based on assessment data
Relate evaluation of effectiveness of care to nursing objectives
	Nursing process in care of the aged:
	  Assessment of the aged client
	  Planning care for the aged
	  Providing care for the aged
	  Evaluating care for the aged

Identify common general pharmacotherapeutic problems in the aged
Identify common problems in administering drugs to the aged
Identify specific side effects of the major drugs when used for the aged
	Nursing responsibility in drug therapy:
	  Effects of aging and drugs
	  Considerations in administration
	  Frequently used drugs
	  Problems in self-administration of drugs by the aged

Table 5-1. *(continued)*
Identify factors related to medication errors among the aged
Describe approaches to reducing the hazards of drug therapy in the aged

Identify activities of interacting, such as observing, listening, and responding verbally and nonverbally Identify and use examples of nondirective techniques to facilitate communication	Supportive interpersonal interaction: 　Basic activities of interaction 　Communication to facilitate expression and understanding
Specify ultimate goal of rehabilitation as independent function within limits of ability Recognize importance of the client's objectives and activity in the rehabilitation process Recognize the importance of fostering independence Demonstrate passive range of motion procedures Describe measures for preventing complications from immobility, deformity, respiratory problems, decubitus ulcers Describe measures for promoting adequate nutrition and elimination in immobile persons Recognize that rehabilitative measures should be incorporated into activities of daily living to the extent possible	Nursing in rehabilitation: 　Rehabilitation goals 　Role of the patient in rehabilitation 　Role of the nurse in rehabilitation 　Preventing complications from immobility 　Fostering independence of aged clients
Define reality orientation Recognize importance of continuity and consistency in reality orientation programs Describe materials commonly used in reality orientation (clocks, etc.) Define milieu therapy as the methodical use of the total environment in treating clients Recognize as the implication of milieu therapy that everything that is done or happens to the person is part of the treatment	Special techniques: 　Reality orientation 　Therapeutic milieu

Table 5-1. (*continued*)
Identify important participants in milieu therapy, including the aged themselves
Recognize physical environmental factors important in milieu therapy
Recognize social environmental factors important in milieu therapy
Recognize daily activities of aged as important factors in milieu therapy

---

Module 4. Nursing in Specific Illnesses and Impairments of the Aged

Objectives	*Content*
Recognize common manifestations of eye problems	Neurologic and behavioral disorders:
Define senile cataract	Visual problems
Define glaucoma	Hearing problems
Identify the objectives of medical treatment of glaucoma	Parkinson's disease
Describe the nursing care for a patient with glaucoma	Organic brain disorders
	Confusion
	Depression

Describe nursing measures appropriate in caring for a blind person
Name and define common causes of deafness in the aged
Identify measures to facilitate communicating with the deaf
Identify common manifestations of Parkinson's disease
Identify objectives of medical treatment of Parkinson's disease
Describe nursing measures commonly used in Parkinson's disease
Identify common causes of confused behavior
Specify the characteristics of confused behavior
Describe nursing care for a confused person
Differentiate delirium, illusion, delusion, and hallucination
Identify the common manifestations of organic brain disorders
Describe nursing care in organic brain disorders
Recognize behavioral changes commonly associated with impending mental problems.
Identify factors predisposing the aged to depression

Table 5-1. (*continued*)

Describe the nurse's role in suicide prevention	Cardiovascular and respiratory disorders: 　Peripheral vascular disease 　Stroke 　Congestive heart failure 　Chronic obstructive lung disease
Recognize common manifestations of peripheral vascular disease	
List precautions in care of the feet in peripheral vascular disease	
Specify common measures for improving and maintaining circulation	
Identify common causes of cerebral vascular accidents	
Describe common psychological and motor concomitants of stroke	
Describe preventive and rehabilitative nursing measures applicable following a stroke	
Describe methods of communicating with an aphasic person	
Recognize the manifestations of left- and right-sided congestive heart failure	
Identify the objectives of medical treatment of congestive heart failure	
Describe preventive and rehabilitative nursing measures for a person with heart disease	
Name the factors related to the development of emphysema	
Define chronic obstructive lung disease (COLD)	
Identify the common manifestations of COLD	
Identify the objectives of treatment of COLD	
Describe palliative and preventive nursing measures appropriate in COLD	
Identify manifestations of CO_2 retention	
Recognize foot problems as a major cause of discomfort in the aged	Other diseases and disorders of aging: 　Skeletomuscular disease and trauma
Name common causes of foot problems	
Define senile osteoporosis	
Recognize the importance of physical activity in treatment of osteoporosis	
Differentiate rheumatoid and osteoarthritis	

Table 5-1. (*continued*)

Identify the objectives of treatment of arthritis	
Recognize factors related to incidence of hip fractures in the aged	
Name the two principal treatments for hip fracture	
Describe the nursing care following internal fixation or hip replacement	
Identify common characteristics of diabetes mellitus in the aged	Diabetes mellitus
Identify common problems of dietary management of diabetes in the aged	
Name the common complications of diabetes	
Differentiate the manifestations of diabetic coma and insulin shock	
Identify common causes of urinary incontinence in the aged	Urinary and bowel elimination disorders
Describe in order the steps in bladder retraining	
Describe nursing measures appropriate in urinary incontinence	
Identify the most common cause and sign of fecal incontinence in the aged	
Identify preventive measures for bowel elimination problems	
Describe in order the steps for bowel retraining	
Define colostomy	
Describe the common care problems associated with colostomy	

6
Undergraduate Education in Gerontic Nursing

Nursing Expertise in Care of the Aged: Need and Deficiency

It seems necessary to preface any treatment of curriculum development in gerontic nursing with a rationale for even including it in the baccalaureate degree programs. In discussing curriculums in some areas of health care—child health care, for example—the fundamental questions might be *how*, or *when*, but not *why*. But when it comes to education programs in the care of the aged population, nursing demands to know *why*. Yet, proclamations from both the public and professional domains of American society declare that the current deficiency in nursing expertise in care of the aged is a serious threat to the welfare of a significant proportion of our society. Nevertheless, there is but meager evidence of any concerted effort on the part of the nursing profession to attack this problem at the fundamental level of preservice nursing education.

The United States Senate Special Committee on Aging focused public attention on deficiencies in research and training in gerontology when it reported, "At present there is a woeful lack of training in the field of aging at all levels and for all types of personnel."[1] The report of the Senate Subcommittee on Long-term Care[2] pointed up deficits in geriatric nursing expertise in particular: "Throughout its investigation the Subcommittee has received much testimony and other evidence which pinpoints the nurse's role in poor patient care." Expert testimony before the subcommittee suggested that problems in the American system of long-term care are a consequence of inadequate numbers of professional nurses prepared in geriatrics.

Nursing itself has spoken to the issue of care for the aged. In 1970, Brown stated:

> . . . the nursing profession like the medical profession has shown relatively little interest in the aged and long-term care to the great detriment of a considerable segment of the population. . . . [3]

As recently as 1975, the American Nurses' Association Report from the Committee on Skilled Nursing Care found it necessary to reiterate the message about the unmet needs of the aged: " . . . An older person seeking assistance finds a dearth of institutions, services, and personnel trained to provide the help that is needed. . . . "[4]

The nursing profession also made positive statements on the importance of nursing care of the aged when, in 1966, the ANA established its Division on Geriatric Nursing Practice, and subsequently devised a system for certification.

But despite these declarations of need and importance, extant data reveal a paucity of baccalaureate level instruction in nursing care of the elderly and cast serious doubt on how much gerontic nursing expertise is considered an important societal need. A 1966 survey of NLN-accredited baccalaureate degree nursing programs by Moses and Lake[5] revealed that only 12 percent of 138 responding schools gave an unqualified "yes" to the question of whether they offered courses with a major emphasis in geriatric nursing. Another survey of 1,072 schools of nursing conducted by Senator Moss in conjunction with the 1969–1973 Senate subcommittee hearings on long-term care, provided additional data consistent with the contention that few schools of nursing emphasize geriatrics to a significant degree.[6]*

More current data on gerontic nursing preparation are now being gathered by the ANA Division on Geriatric Nursing Practice, but there is no evidence yet available to contradict the assumption that instruction in nursing care of the aged remains notably lacking from the education of registered nurses in the United States. This assumption is supported by the fact that gerontic nursing is still not included in the nurse licensure examination. The significance of this fact should not be overlooked, because, first of all, the licensure examination is a message from the nursing profession about itself: inclusion of a content area in a licensure examination constitutes a stamp of approval and reflects a reciprocal relationship with curriculum development.

Arguments Supporting Curriculum Development

Although the dearth of instruction in gerontic nursing has persisted, nursing has not been without a cadre of advocates for including it in baccalaureate degree programs.

Certainly the most frequently cited basis for concern about health care for the aged is the sheer number of aging people. The fact that the aged population is increasing in absolute size, in proportional size, and in age (the 75 + subgroup is expanding rapidly) has caught the attention of public and professional groups including nursing.

There are, in addition, other variables that should enter into a rational decision, regardless of how many old people there are. The nursing literature reveals that among a variety of such other factors which are a source of concern to nursing educators, that of attitude toward the aged is ubiquitous. Attitude has probably been talked about and measured (at least purported to have been

*It should be noted that the report of the subcommittee refers to " . . . all 1,072 schools of nursing." It is not clear what population is designated by that phrase, since NLN data for 1971 reveal 1,363 basic programs preparing registered nurses.

measured) more often than all other variables combined. The literature reflects a general belief that negative attitudes about nursing held by both students and practitioners of nursing are a barrier to quality care of the aged, and thus learning experiences with the aged to alter these attitudes are a necessity.

Other factors cited as indicating a need for formal gerontic nursing instruction include: the high incidence of chronic disease among the elderly and/or their disproportionately high use of health care facilities;[7][8][9] the emergence of gerontology and the subsequent availability of knowledge about the elderly;[10] legislation which has resulted in an increase in the number of facilities for the aged and the consequent increase in the numbers of registered nurses needed to care for the aged; and, finally, the distinctiveness of the content and practice of gerontic nursing. It seems reasonable that the sum of these factors should point up the need to teach gerontic nursing. Yet, overall, the impact on educational decisions regarding preparation for gerontic nursing has been negligible, possibly because these factors are so diverse. Perhaps collectively they could be an effective stimulus for change. In other words, it may be that nursing needs to ask, "What answers to the educationally important questions are inherent in these diverse factors?"

Arguments Supporting the Need for Gerontic Nursing Preparation

We have proposed four questions below. We believe that the correct answers to these questions will logically show the importance of including gerontic nursing in baccalaureate degree programs.

What Is Known about Health Care for the Aging?

The development of gerontology and the expansion of knowledge about the aged provide the answer to this question. A secondary question then becomes, "Do we know if the aged differ from others we care for?" Yes, they do differ in some respects, and the nature of the differences is beginning to be known through our expanding knowledge of humans as they age.

Undergraduate Education

Do Nurses Need to Know It?

Rephrased, this question might be stated, "Do the differences of the aged require different nursing capabilities?"* There is no consensus on this point. In their survey of geriatrics in the baccalaureate nursing curriculum, Moses and Lake (1966) found opposing views.[12] Some respondents took the view that " '. . . geriatrics is a distinct content and practice area which is specialized.' This view holds that nursing the aged does require knowledge about aging."

Others negate the usefulness of a "specialized" approach to geriatric nursing, considering it rather as a part of "total nursing." In this view, "total nursing" encompasses all there is to be known about nursing anyone; thus, nursing the aged does not have any particular requirements that require special educational attention. We take the opposite position.

Can It Be Taught?

The answer to this question is implicit in the literature. Obviously, some in nursing believe the answer is yes. We propose that if nursing the aged comprises some set of learned capabilities with general applicability to the aged, then at least some components can probably be taught. It remains to be demonstrated whether a component such as attitude can be taught within the constraints of a course or two in nursing education programs.

Which Nurses Should Be Taught?

Because of the numbers of aging, the high incidence of disease, and the disproportionately high use of health care facilities by the aged, the probability is high that any nurse will encounter a goodly number of aged clients. This being so, it seems necessary

---

*The term *capability* is used in the sense proposed by Gagne and Briggs[11]: learned capabilities are the outcome of instruction that makes possible varieties of human performance. They include information, cognitive skills and strategies, motor skills, and attitudes.

that preservice preparation for all nurses include the development of capabilities for caring for the aged.

In summary, we propose that, given our present state of knowledge, an affirmative answer to each of these questions is supported by both data and logic. These affirmative answers, in turn, clearly lead to a decision that gerontic nursing should be included in the basic preparation of all nursing students at the baccalaureate degree level. While this decision is based on what, at present, seems best for nursing students, it does not preclude the need for sound research to test the assumptions upon which it is based.

Some Factors to Be Considered in Gerontic Nursing Curriculums

Nursing the aged, or gerontic nursing, was defined in Chapter 2 as a health service that incorporates generic nursing methods and specialized knowledge about the aged to establish conditions within the client and/or within the environment that will:

1. Increase health-conducive behaviors in the aged
2. Minimize and compensate for health-prejudical losses and impairments of aging
3. Provide comfort and sustenance through the distressing and debilitating events of aging, including dying and death
4. Facilitate the diagnosis, palliation, and treatment of disease(s) in the aged

Nursing competence obviously incorporates capabilities that are not specific to nursing and were acquired long before the individual entered a nursing education program. The task of nursing education is to build on these capabilities additional capabilities that are seen by educators as requisites for nursing. Certain capabilities are recognized as being common to all nursing, but they require special adaptation to the needs of older persons. The uniqueness of gerontic nursing seems to be primarily in the use of the information—that is, the facts, concepts,

Undergraduate Education

and principles of gerontology—to obtain the best fit of judgements, aims, and actions to aged clients.

The nursing profession does not know when it has achieved good gerontic nursing because nurses have not yet found a consistent way to measure nursing effectiveness objectively. Educators must, therefore, teach what they *think* is best for students to know. Meanwhile, nurses must continue to ponder questions about competencies for nursing, and, more than that, seek ways to ultimately test out some answers.

Assuming that there is something that can reasonably be called gerontic nursing, and that we do know something about what it probably is, there are a number of areas to consider if we are going to teach it. Overall, the instructional task at the baccalaureate degree level is to select what seem the *most* crucial and widely applicable elements of gerontic nursing and incorporate them into a required introductory course. Selecting the content of instruction may well be the most critical decision that is made in any course design. Yet it seems that all too often preoccupation with instructional methods has caused educators to lose sight of the importance of course content and disregard rigorous and objective measurement of the students' mastery of the content. Therefore, a brief consideration of some crucial points about instructional development seems warranted.

Instructional Objectives

A fundamental task in designing any course is to identify what it is that students should be able to do after they have completed the course. A word of warning: this task should not be equated with the educational ritual called "writing objectives." Time wasted in conjuring up new verbs for "behavioral" objectives could probably be better spent on a detailed description of a competent nurse, on a careful selection and analysis of course content, and on the construction of reliable and valid tools for measuring mastery of the content. High quality instruction can happen in the absence of explicit "behavioral" objectives, as they are too often formulated, but it cannot happen in the absence of content. What is implied here is that general statements defining the broad content areas should be included in the course of instruction, along with a statement of what the student is expected to do with that content. An example of a first step in this direction is provided by the following statement on competencies at the baccalaureate degree level in gerontic nursing.

Expected competencies in gerontic nursing at the baccalaureate degree level. At the completion of the required instructional program in gerontic nursing at the baccalaureate degree level, it is expected that students will be able to demonstrate mastery of:

1. The basic tenets of selected theories of aging
2. Characteristics of common social and psychological developmental events of aging
3. Major changes associated with aging in physiological functioning in the absence of overt disease
4. Changes associated with aging in response to pathological conditions common among the aged
5. Changes associated with aging in response to measures aimed at promoting, maintaining, and restoring health, for example, exercise, drug therapy
6. The interactive effects of functional age changes and/or multiple disease conditions
7. Resources appropriate for utilization or referral by nurses

The student should be able to use knowledge in direct care of the aged clients to:

1. Search for and recognize evidence of health deficits, functional decrements, distress, and disease in aged clients
2. Formulate achievable nursing goals that are congruent with the goals of clients to increase health, cope with losses, provide comfort and sustenance, and manage disease; and establish the internal and external conditions necessary to achieve these goals
3. Select and execute nursing methods in a manner that assures safety and maximizes effectiveness

The student should be able to use knowledge in indirect care of the aged to:

1. Communicate knowledge about the aged
2. Direct and instruct other levels of nursing personnel
3. Communicate effectively in written and oral nursing records, reports, referrals, and consultations
4. Teach, advise, and counsel the "significant others" of aged clients
5. Make appropriate referrals

The student should be able to verify and expand his or her knowledge by:

1. Searching for relationships between the observed behavior of aged clients and the theoretical and hypothetical constructs of gerontology
2. Locating and using appropriate source materials about the aged

Instructional Content

Once the broad areas of competency have been formulated, further specification of content is vital. Content coverage and emphasis have an effect on student achievement. Table 6-1 presents a proposed content outline. (See Appendix A for a sample of a content analysis guide and a content summary for two different lessons.)

Table 6-1.
Content Outline for an Introductory Course in Gerontic Nursing at the Baccalaureate Degree Level

	Module 1. Gerontic Nursing: An Orientation and Overview
Lesson 1.	Contemporary cultural context of aging in the United States
	demography of aging "old" as socioculturally defined societal attitudes
Lesson 2.	Multidisciplinary approaches to the phenomenon of aging
	gerontology geriatrics gerontic nursing

Table 6-1. (*continued*)

Module 2. Dimensions of Aging

Lesson 1. Biological developmental events

    general physiological changes
    tissue changes
    organ and organ system changes
    pathological changes

Lesson 2. Sociological developmental events

    work role changes
    economic changes
    social relationship changes
    status and power changes

Lesson 3. Psychological developmental events

    cognitive changes
    motivational, time orientation, goal changes
    affective changes
    self-concept changes

Lesson 4. Selected theories and views of aging

    cellular theories
    activity vs disengagement theories
    developmental views

Module 3. Nursing Focuses for Health-conducive Behavior

Lesson 1. Personal care and safety

    prevention of injury
    personal appearance and grooming
    activities of daily living
    comfort

Lesson 2. Physical fitness

    sleep
    exercise
    nutrition
    health screening

Lesson 3. Personal needs

    cognitive stimulation
    social interaction
    sexuality

Undergraduate Education

Table 6-1. (continued)
  leisure—recreation activity
  useful roles
  shelter—personal space

Module 4. Nursing Focuses in Functional Loss and Disability

Lesson 1. Sensory loss and perceptual impairment

  vision
  hearing
  taste/smell
  pain/tactile

Lesson 2. Loss of mobility

  disuse phenomena
  neurologic impairment
  musculoskeletal disorders

Lesson 3. Pain and illness

  hospitalization/institutionalization
  drug therapy
  rehabilitation

Lesson 4. Dying and death

  stages of dying
  needs of the dying

Module 5. Nursing Focuses in Psychosocial Impairments

Lesson 1. Organic brain disorders

  acute brain syndrome
  chronic brain syndrome

Lesson 2. Functional disorders

  paranoid states
  psychophysiologic reactions
  depressive reactions

Lesson 3. Transient situational reactions

  grief
  loneliness
  anxiety

Module 6. Nursing Focuses in Chronic Disease

Lesson 1. Diabetes

  manifestations in the aged
  management
  complications

Table 6-1. (*continued*)

Lesson 2. Gastrointestinal disorders

    functional disorders
    cancer
    drug therapy

Lesson 3. Cardiovascular/pulmonary disorders

    congestive heart failure
    hypertension
    peripheral vascular diseases
    chronic obstructive lung disease
    drug therapy

Lesson 4. Genitourinary disorders

    urinary incontinence
    urinary tract infections and obstructions
    drug therapy

Module 7. Gerontic Nursing Methods and Resources

Lesson 1. Nursing process

    assessment
    planning
    implementation
    evaluation

Lesson 2. Community resources

    local
    state
    national

One kind of content that seems particularly important in gerontic nursing is that provided by the nursing practice laboratory—learning experiences involving direct patient contact. For example, including in the laboratory experiences a representative sample of the aged population might help change stereotypical attitudes toward gerontic nursing. The sample should include the healthy aged, the ill aged, those in the community, and those in institutions. All that may be accomplished by contact with one or two patients in the same setting would be the exchange of old stereotypes for new ones based on the idiosyncrasies of one or two clients.

Ideally, the instructional content in client settings should incorporate the recognition and interpretation of evidence of health-related needs in the aged, the selection of appropriate nursing aims, the establishment of appropriate conditions to achieve these aims, and judgments about the success of the nursing actions employed. Thus, concern with the content of this part of the learning experience is a part of the overall concern with the content of instruction.

Instructional Means

If the *content* of instruction has not always captured the interest of nursing educators, the *means* of instruction surely has. Unfortunately, educational literature in gerontic nursing is characterized more by enthusiastic anecdotal reports than by research, and the research is often fatally flawed. A common error is to find a pretest-posttest design in which there are no direct comparisons between experimental and control groups. For example, if pretest-posttest comparison shows no difference for the control group, but does show a significant difference for the experimental group, the conclusion is drawn that the experimental treatment is the better of the two.

Clearly, systematic research is needed on decisions about instruction. If we follow one rule-of-thumb about methods, perhaps the view of Rothkopf[13] (and many others) will help, i.e., that the essential component of learning from reading is active cognitive processing. The instructor may be well advised to define what it is she wants the student to learn and then select whatever methods and strategies will induce the learner to engage in deep cognitive processing.

Measurement of instruction outcomes. How do we measure the outcomes of instruction? If the content has been selected because nursing educators think it is important for nursing students to know, then it is reasonable to assume that reliable and valid measures of how well the job has been accomplished are necessary.

Of course it would be desirable to require that nursing teachers have formal preparation in test construction and principles of measurement. Alternatives are to have a well-prepared resource person on the nursing faculty or to fully utilize resources outside the nursing education unit, for example, other instructional service units within the institution.

In one project to measure instructional outcomes, the nurse authors and educational psychologists collaborated in developing an item-writing system. The nurse authors assembled the instructional materials for each course. They read the materials carefully and highlighted the important content items with a felt-tipped pen. These items were developed by the nurse authors and the psychologists in the following sequence:

1. Test item constructed from material by nurse authors and their assistants
2. Test item critiqued by one member of the educational psychology team
3. Test item revised by nurse authors
4. Final review and approval of all test items by nurse authors
5. Field testing of items by administrative personnel to resident nursing students
6. Items revised on basis of field-test data

Though implementation of such an elaborate system may be desirable, it is not always feasible. However, given that not all nurse educators are likely to have had formal courses in test construction, some useful techniques were found that are applicable in most any situation.

An item-writing manual* with concise summaries and illustrations of item-writing principles will provide guidelines for both writing and critiquing items. A common fault in item sampling is letting the ease of turning a content item into a test item determine what content will be covered in a test. To avoid this pitfall, the project director divided the material into short segments a few pages in length, underlined the crucial information

---

*The manual that proved useful to the nurses in the project discussed here was *Improving the Classroom Test: A Manual of Test Construction Procedures for Classroom Teachers*, Albany: The University of the State of New York, The Education Department, Bureau of Examination and Testing, 1959.

in each segment of text, and targetted the important content with test items. In this way, content is included in the test on the basis of its importance, rather than how easily it lends itself to test item-writing.

Another check on content sampling can be done by extending the content analysis technique previously described (see Appendix A). Test items can be classified according to the kind of content they target: suppositions, concepts, etc. For example, an overabundance of items in the "Facts" column and a scarcity in the "Concepts" and "Principles" columns can be graphically displayed.

Options for Instruction. Many areas of information need to be considered when planning the basic preparation required in gerontic nursing, and the amount of time that can be allotted to one course is, of necessity, limited. If the nursing profession is committed to recruiting nurses to care for the aged, what can it do to nourish interest that is sparked in an introductory course? One answer is to provide courses beyond the required course in gerontic nursing.

In summary, a number of factors should be considered by those who design gerontic nursing education programs. The aims of instruction must be clarified, not only in the mind of the teacher, but in the minds of the students as well. While decisions about instructional methods are important, at present no evidence indicates that any *one* educational innovation will guarantee a generally marked improvement in learning. Nurse educators should, therefore, at least try to separate fact from fancy in decisions about instructional means. In the realm of attitude learning, providing both successful experience with the aged and appropriate nursing role models deserves careful consideration.

While the content of instruction seems to have received less emphasis than the means of instruction, closer attention to content is warranted by research showing that students tend to learn content that is covered better than content that is not covered.

Finally, measurement of learning outcomes is also an important component of instruction. Improvement in the quality of nursing care of the aged obviously cannot be effected by good intentions alone. If we believe that gerontic nursing involves capabilities that can be learned and, further, that the well-being of a significant portion of our society depends on nurses learning those capabilities, then it is important that we not only design and implement instruction to foster that learning but also that we develop reliable and valid means for measuring the success of our efforts.

7
Graduate Education in Gerontic Nursing

The objective of basic nursing education is to prepare students to care for persons with disease or disability and, in baccalaureate programs, the scope of care also includes health promotion and maintenance. Graduate study prepares nurses for clinical specialization and to function in expanded roles. These roles require of nurses not only skills in caring for persons undergoing complex therapies in acute and intensive care; and health promotion and maintenance, including teaching, counseling, advising, and demonstration techniques; but also knowledge and skill in the sophisticated techniques of health assessment. These assessment skills are used in planning, implementing, and evaluating nursing care. Graduate programs prepare nurses to fulfill the leadership roles of teaching, administration, and research, in addition to the specialized clinical competencies.

The purpose of this chapter is to provide an overview of possible programs of graduate studies designed to prepare nurses for positions in gerontic nursing, and to provide some guidelines for the development of graduate education in gerontic nursing.

While it is hoped that the information will have nationwide usefulness to people designing programs, specific illustrations have been drawn from work at The Pennsylvania State University from 1971 to 1976 to illustrate how the programs may be organized and offered, as well as the resources that may be available for the conduct of the programs. We intend to examine the nature of graduate education in aging and gerontology and then to discuss graduate education in gerontic nursing. In addition, we will attempt to describe the resources that are available in this field of nursing and to provide examples of course development at the graduate level.

Graduate Education in Aging Within the Social Sciences, edited by Rose E. Kushner and Marion E. Bunch,[1] has been used for the design of graduate education programs in aging. The guidelines it offers were designed by an ad hoc committee on professional training and curriculum development, which was appointed in 1961 by the psychology and social sciences section of the Gerontological Society. While this book emphasizes doctoral programs in social gerontology, the authors recognize that master's degree programs are also needed to prepare people to fill various kinds of positions, particularly positions in the service professions.

The purpose of graduate programs in gerontic nursing is to educate highly qualified professional nurses to provide expert nursing and health services to the elderly population. Graduates of these programs will be expected to take the lead in surveying societal needs and in developing nursing skills, knowledge, and practice competencies in light of apparent needs. It is also expected that the graduates will be able to demonstrate collaborative and effective interaction with nurses and other health professions and disciplines in effecting changes in nursing practice and the delivery of health care.

What Is Graduate Education in Nursing?

Graduate education in nursing has come to mean increasingly the specialization in nursing practice, and preparation for research, teaching, and administration. The aim of specialization in professional practice is to prepare the nurse to be skilled in meeting the nursing care needs of selected patients. The nurse must learn to give attention to patient welfare, safety, satisfaction, and efficacy of treatment. This preparation is based on knowledge of the scientific principles guiding nursing practice, with consideration of the moral, ethical, and legal aspects of health care.

Graduate preparation is essential to prepare highly skilled nurse practitioners or clinicians to assume responsibility for patients undergoing complex medical treatment. Practitioners must be prepared for the independent and interdependent activities designed to promote and maintain health in the primary or ambulatory care setting. Nursing faculty must be prepared to teach in schools of nursing, and must have advanced preparation for professional practice and curriculum design, course development, and educational technology, and for in-service and continuing education programs. Nurses must be prepared to administer nursing services in hospitals and community health agencies and to study problems in nursing using the scientific method for the improvement of patient care, nursing education, and the organization of nursing services. Application of this knowledge is done in a practicum under the supervision of nursing faculty.

Aims and Objectives

The academic objectives of graduate education in nursing are to:

1. Develop skill in use of information resources and in the synthesis and integration of existing knowledge
2. Advance knowledge in the field through research
3. Prepare for specific occupational functions of advanced nursing practice in clinical, educational, or executive settings

The professional objectives of graduate preparation in nursing are to:

1. Afford students opportunities to develop greater proficiency in nursing and health care

2. Promote clinical research and writing in nursing and health care
3. Prepare students to confront problems in health care services with the aim of developing effective solutions for conflict, ambiguities, and questions encountered in practice

The graduate school of The Pennsylvania State University recognizes different career purposes in two types of advanced degrees, academic and professional. The graduate nursing student whose goal is a career in education, research, or administration may choose the Master of Science program. The Master of Science (M.S.) is an academic degree awarded for fulfillment of courses stressing scholarship and research. To support individual career aims, the Master of Science candidate has a choice of functional options, either teaching or administration. It should be emphasized that the Master of Science degree does not prepare for a career in research but only provides the basis for further study at the doctoral level should the student desire to prepare for a career in nursing research. The Master of Nursing (M.N.) is the professional degree conferred upon successful completion of courses emphasizing the use of applied science in the solution of health care problems.

Behavioral Objectives of the Program Leading to the
Master of Nursing Degree

At the completion of the graduate program, the student should have a defined role as a clinical specialist in a specific area of nursing. The student should be able to:
1. Give specialized nursing care and play an instrumental role in aiding individuals and families in meeting health care and nursing needs
2. Apply new knowledge in the specialty area to implement innovations in nursing practice
3. Accept responsibility for participating in continuing education programs in the specialty area
4. Think critically, creatively, and independently to effect changes in the specialty area

Graduate Education

The student should have increased knowledge of the physical, behavioral, and social sciences of sufficient depth and perspective to allow for systematic study of specific concepts and their application to nursing practice, as demonstrated by ability to:

1. Identify and define the concept (s)
2. Interpret or explain alternate solutions, including the rationale for each
3. Draw inferences and support conclusion(s)
4. Perform in a clinically competent manner

The student should have the ability to demonstrate by independent study and to present in a systematic and orderly fashion, the results of clinical studies by:

1. Stating and defining the clinical problem
2. Describing the approach used in studying the problem
3. Synthesizing the data collected
4. Giving a valid interpretation of the data

The student should have the ability to assist others to understand and interpret facts and inferences of the basic concepts of health care, as demonstrated by:

1. Teaching individual patients and families, or groups of patients and families
2. Participating with personnel from other disciplines in cooperative research endeavors

Behavioral Objectives of the Program Leading to the
Master of Science Degree

At the completion of the graduate program, the student should have increased knowledge of the physical, behavioral, and social sciences of sufficient depth and perspective to allow for systematic study of specific concepts and their application to nursing practice, as demonstrated by ability to:

1. Identify and define the concept(s)
2. Interpret or explain alternate solutions, including the rationale for each

3. Draw inferences and support conclusion(s)
4. Perform in a clinically competent manner

The student should have the initiative and ability to use research methodology to improve the practice of nursing, as demonstrated by ability to:

1. Redefine, reorder, or identify existing or new knowledge pertinent to nursing practice
2. Develop approaches for the delivery of nursing care to the patient
3. Identify and solve problems that are barriers to efficient and therapeutic health care

The student should have the ability to demonstrate by independent study, and to present in a systematic and orderly fashion, the results of findings using:

1. A statement and definition of the problem identified
2. A description of the methodological approach used
3. A synthesis of the data collected
4. A valid interpretation of the data

The student should have the ability and initiative to formulate and subject to empirical test and inference concepts and theories that contribute to nursing knowledge using:

1. Definitive abstractions
2. Synthesis and operational definitions
3. Theory construction based upon testable hypotheses

The student should have the ability to assist others to understand and interpret facts and inferences of the basic concepts of health care as demonstrated by:

1. Teaching individual patients and families or groups of patients and families
2. Teaching in a formal academic setting
3. Participating with personnel from other disciplines in cooperative research endeavors

Planning Graduate Programs

Very early in the process of making a decision to establish a graduate program in gerontic nursing, consultation should be sought from the National League for Nursing (NLN), Department of Baccalaureate and Higher Degree Programs. The timing for seeking consultation will depend on a particular faculty; some will desire consultation before and some after they have developed a plan. In any event, the faculty will need two NLN guides to use in their deliberations: the *Criteria for the Appraisal of Baccalaureate and Higher Degree Programs in Nursing*,[2] and the *Policies and Procedures of Accreditation for Programs in Nursing Education*.[3] The criteria were developed to assist schools in developing and improving educational programs and are used by the accrediting body for the appraisal of educational programs. Criteria are provided for the organization and administration of an academic unit, students, faculty, curriculum, resources, facilities, and services.

Another important source of information on the establishment of graduate programs is the Council of Graduate Schools in the United States.* The Council notes that the quality of the professors involved is of utmost importance in the establishment of a sound program. Professors should be scholars in their fields (usually evidenced by the doctoral degree), and should have proven capacity for teaching and research.[4] The program may require one or two years and should consist of a coherent sequence of lectures, seminars, and independent studies or investigations at the master's level, which will assist the student to acquire an introduction to the mastery of knowledge, creative scholarship, and research in the field. A thesis and a rigorous comprehensive examination are usually required for a master of arts or a master of science program. The professional master's degrees vary somewhat in requirements from the academic degrees.

*Address inquiries to: The President, Council of Graduate Schools in the United States, 1 Dupont Circle, Washington, D.C. Available booklets are: *The Master's Degree*, *The Doctor of Philosophy Degree*, and *The Doctor's Degree in Professional Fields*.

Once a decision is made—based upon a documented need and demand for the program, availability of faculty, sufficient financial support, and academic facilities (space, library, computer, etc.)—that an academic unit in nursing should develop a graduate program in nursing, a proposal must be developed for approval by the graduate school, faculty senate, or other academic body. The persons or committee designated to undertake this task will need to establish communication with the group empowered to approve the proposal. This is usually done through the administration of the Graduate School. It is helpful to obtain copies of recently approved program proposals of other academic units of the university. Guidelines provided by these units will help the faculty focus on the program requirements and issues and, in the long run, will save them time in developing the proposal.

For example, in one university, the request for approval of graduate programs requires first the justification of nursing as a major field. It may appear unusual or unnecessary to nursing faculty to have to justify graduate education in nursing since it has been in existence for many years. But university faculty outside and, at times, inside health science centers may not grant nursing the serious consideration it deserves. Nursing faculty should look on this request for justification as an opportunity to educate a very important segment of their public and to establish relationships within the university community for collaboration in research, teaching, and community service.

The nursing faculty may select courses from the university as support courses as well as propose offering courses in nursing no other academic unit is prepared to offer. Some courses in nursing may be cross-listed with those offered in other departments. In addition, some nursing courses may be suitable for non-nursing students. As nursing students need and benefit from other university courses, so do other students benefit from nursing courses.

The approving body may want to know why it should offer graduate education in nursing. This question may be answered by describing the number of graduate programs in the state and other programs in neighboring states.

Finally, the faculty will need to specify their long-range goals and plans for the future together with time tables and at least five-year projections for the proposed program. Brochures and other descriptive materials will need to be prepared for recruitment after the program is approved by the graduate council or other similar body in the univeristy.

Issues in Graduate Education

First are the issues pertaining to the field of aging studies. What type of degree should be offered in a graduate education program in aging? Should it be a Ph.D. in gerontology, in social gerontology, or in a social science discipline with a major in aging? The principal differences among the objectives of the three programs that prepare for these three degrees reflect differences in the breadth or scope of the sciences in which graduate students would be expected to achieve scholarship and competence. Questions about the student's future career goals arise: Will his training be too broad and of insufficient depth to prepare him for research in a particular area should he aspire to the Ph.D. in gerontology?

A related issue concerns specialization in nursing and appropriate titles for specialists within the subfields of nursing. The American Nurses' Association has officially recognized five areas of specialization in nursing: medical-surgical nursing; maternal and child health nursing; psychiatric and mental health nursing; public health and community health nursing; and geriatric nursing—more recently changed to gerontological nursing.

Another issue concerns whether the emphasis in graduate programs should be on old age, with a problem-centered approach, or the life-span, developmental approach. In the literature, psychologists appear to support the life-span approach to a greater extent than do representatives of other disciplines. The professionals, of necessity, support a problem-centered approach. Both approaches are probably essential in that each stage of life has its particular crises and problems. But while particular kinds of problems occur in old age, it is also essential to understand antecedents of change, as well as continuities through time. These can best be understood through the life-span, developmental approach.

Organization and Administration of a Graduate Program

A graduate program designed to prepare nurses in gerontic nursing should subscribe to the general philosophy and educational philosophy set forth by the academic unit in nursing, the graduate school, and the university in which the program is located. It should be organized in such a manner that interdisciplinary study in aging is possible and experiences in various human services serving the aged population can be arranged.

Consideration should be given to developing policies that will be used to govern and guide the students. Areas in which policies are usually needed include clinical assignment, travel, equipment, grading, course registration, liability insurance, theses, clinical papers, and so on.

In the organization and administration of a graduate program in a particular specialization there should be a professor-in-charge or some appropriate academic officer who will be responsible to the associate or assistant dean in charge of graduate programs in the nursing unit. The responsibilities should include some combination of the following activities, depending upon the structure of the academic unit:

1. Monitoring the quality and effectiveness of the program
2. Considering the views and suggestions of the faculty specialization groups on changes, innovations, developments, and implementation of programs
3. Assisting in the recruitment and selection of faculty and supporting personnel
4. Preparing reports and descriptive materials pertaining to the program, i.e., university senate, bulletins, NLN accreditation
5. Chairing a committee on the program

6. Seeking funds for support of components of the program, i.e., research, teaching improvement projects, fellowships, traineeships, etc.
7. Preparing an annual report for the person responsible for graduate programs

In addition, there needs to be supporting personnel, including secretarial personnel and an administrative assistant either for this program or for the graduate program as a whole, depending on the size of the various units.

Facilities

The resources, facilities, and services required for graduate programs in gerontic nursing are similar to those required in other nursing programs and in other disciplines and professional areas that provide services for the aged.

The availability and adequacy of facilities, particularly clinical facilities, need to be described. Attention must be given to library and research facilities, laboratories and supporting services, and space for seminars and instruction, as well as to desk space for faculty, assistants, and graduate students. Not to be overlooked is space for administrative personnel. Space is essential for the image the graduate program presents to prospective and enrolled students, the university community, and the public.

Ideally, there should be a center or a similar organization in which can take place communication, forums, and seminars comprised of faculty in several disciplines who are conducting research in the various facets of aging. Students should have an opportunity to work with both students and faculty in other departments of the university on the common problems of aging.

A variety of clinical settings may be used for teaching, including hospitals, clinics, ambulatory services, nursing homes and residential treatment centers, and community agencies, as well as the traditional health care agencies. In many of these facilities, however, innovations are needed to improve learning experiences of both graduate and undergraduate students. Perhaps one solution would be the development of a large number of demonstration centers with faculty assuming some responsibility for the administration of these units. The difficulties of this approach, however, pose an important dilemma for nursing.

The Clinical Teaching Setting

If clinical settings are to be used, guidelines for protecting patient welfare should be given consideration in planning educational programs. In order to provide for quality control and maintenance of high standards of nursing care, the following guidelines are suggested:

1. The nurse-patient relationship is established when a nursing student is assigned to care for a patient. The nurse legally owes a special duty of care to the assigned patients. The legal status of the student is the same as that of a registered nurse. Graduate students should take a course in the legal aspects of nursing, if they have not had the course in undergraduate school.

2. The ANA Standards of Nursing Practice provide an authoritative statement by which the quality of general nursing practice may be measured. In addition, the Divisions of Practice have developed Standards of Maternal and Child Health Nursing Practice; Psychiatric and Mental Health Nursing Practice; Geriatric Nursing Practice; Community Health Nursing Practice; and Medical-Surgical Nursing Practice. These may be used in conjunction with the generic Standards of Nursing Practice or an individual instructor may develop Standards of Nursing Practice for a specific course. When these specific Standards of Nursing Practice are in use, a copy should be filed with the professor-in-charge of the graduate curriculum, a copy filed with the course outline, and a copy provided for the director of the nursing service where students are receiving their experience.

3. Faculty and students are responsible and accountable for the quality of nursing care provided. All persons involved should participate in evaluation of nursing care at the end of each clinical assignment.

4. The occurence of an injury, or deviation from expected performance, or an untoward incident should be described in

triplicate form within 24 hours and copies provided to the appropriate professor-in-charge of the graduate curriculum, and the dean or head of the Department of Nursing. In addition, the necessary forms should be completed and filed as required by the agency in which the incident occurred.

5. All persons are responsible for their negligent acts. Nursing students must meet the same standard of performance as the registered nurse. If, for any reason, a student feels that she cannot provide safe and efficient care, she should notify the persons to whom she is responsible, beginning with the most immediate person, i.e., the student should tell the instructor, who informs the professor-in-charge, who notifies the dean or head of the department, and so on. Every person must have recourse to someone in the organization so that the patient's welfare will be safeguarded and the nurse or nursing student be protected from accusations of malpractice or professional negligence.

6. The general rights of patients and families which all nurses and nursing students should observe include courtesy, nonjudgmental treatment, and considerate care. If a patient does not wish a student to provide care, or refuses a treatment, then the patient's wishes must be respected. It is also expected that courtesy, respect, and nonjudgmental attitudes will apply to all people, personnel, and all nursing and medical staffs.

7. The guidelines provided by the university committee on the use of human subjects in thesis and clinical papers should be followed.

Faculty

In determining how many faculty members are needed for a new graduate program, normal teaching load is used to measure the extent to which graduate instruction and thesis supervision can be undertaken by the existing faculty.

An estimate of the present graduate enrollment and the enrollment predicted by a specified time period—usually five years—will need to be made. Also needed is a list of the current upper-division courses appropriate for both undergraduate and graduate students, as well as a list of the upper-division and graduate courses and practices that will be used to maintain the integrity of graduate courses.

Any recent regional or state studies, national surveys, and studies and statements by nursing organizations may help to document the faculty needs. The shortage of well-qualified faculty is still acute in most areas, as are specialists in nursing and persons prepared for administrative roles and those prepared for an extended role in primary care.

The strengths and weaknesses of the nursing faculty will need to be examined with particular attention to faculty size, training, "inbreeding," research output, interest in graduate education, ability to assist with theses and dissertations, and evidence of its national reputation.

Ideally, faculty members should have doctoral preparation in an area related to aging and nursing. Recruitment efforts should be directed toward a faculty with at least two-thirds of the members holding doctoral degrees and graduate faculty status in the university. To implement quality graduate programs requires a strong nursing faculty with university-level competence and credentials, as well as technical nursing competence.

Nursing faculty, as other faculty in the university, are expected to engage in a combination of activities such as were outlined by Gaff and Wilson:

1. Classroom teaching activities—lecturing, leading discussions, suggesting reading references, making assignments.
2. Preparatory classroom activities—reading assigned books, preparing notes, constructing reading lists, devising assignments, preparing laboratory demonstrations, securing equipment for studio classes.
3. Associated housekeeping activities—taking roll, making problem sets, preparing quizzes and examinations, reading and grading quizzes and examinations, reading term papers, evaluating class projects.
4. Course-planning activities—reconsidering the needs and interests of students, the state of the field and its relation to society, reviewing possible textbooks, planning course sequences.
5. Out-of-class teaching activities—talking with students about classroom discussions, clarifying assignments, helping students plan and prepare term papers or projects, holding paper or exami-

nation conferences, discussing intellectual matters with students, helping students learn how to study, supervising independent study.

6. Advising and counseling activities—discussing students' vocational aims and plans, advising about academic programs, discussing students' problems, gathering relevant information from other faculty or administrators, acting to help students with difficulties, writing letters of recommendation.

7. Student extracurricular activities—advising student organizations, chaperoning dances, attending student social functions, discussing campus issues with student groups.

8. Activities concerned with keeping up-to-date in one's field—reading books and professional journals in one's specialty, reading in related fields, reading about general cultural developments, attending professional meetings, corresponding with colleagues elsewhere, writing for books, articles, and papers, ordering books for the library.

9. Activities to become informed about campus issues—talking with colleagues both in and outside of one's department, discussing issues with members of various committees, talking with administrators, reading school newspapers, reading memos, position papers, or planning documents.

10. Departmental governance activities—attending department meetings, serving on department committees, writing memos, proposals, or position papers.

11. Division, college, or university governance activities—same as above.

12. Graduate education activities—selecting students from applicants, recommending financial assistance for students, preparing, administering, and evaluating graduate examinations, serving on thesis committees, securing jobs for graduates.

13. Research and scholarly activities—writing proposals, administering funds, supervising assistance, conducting research, preparing reports, writing papers, speaking to colleagues, consulting with other schools, government, or business.[5]

This list of activities is further increased by clinical teaching. Clinical courses in nursing are different from other university courses because the amount of time spent in the clinical areas or the community is in addition to time spent in student advising, committee work, and community service or professional organization activities. Time spent in class preparation, examination grading, and assignments often leaves little time for research, writing, and professional service commitments.

A major unresolved problem in nursing education at the present time is how to plan so that undergraduate and graduate students can have suitable learning experiences in organized nursing and community services.

Interest in giving formal structure to the close relationship between nursing education and nursing service grows out of the need to provide exemplary nursing services to people. If the most up-to-date theoretical knowledge of the nursing faculty was combined with the real-life experiences of a selected well-qualified nursing service staff, an ideal learning environment for students and exemplary service for patients would result. One such possibility for achieving this is the organization of a facility or place where graduate students could design and evaluate various theories about patient care and where experimentation and research directed toward the improvement of services could occur.

Problems in designing such an organization are caused by the nature of nursing services, which require a constant vigilance, 24 hours a day, 365 days a year, and the nature of university teaching, which combines a variety of activities, only a few of which are organized on a time schedule. The work of the nurse in nursing services has traditionally been organized into 8-hour shifts. Top-echelon nurses are administratively responsible for 24-hour periods. In some instances (in outpatient and in-service education units, for example) work can be organized into shorter time periods. Consultation functions of the nurse specialists may be provided to both patients and staff in brief time segments, but these activities may also be organized in such a way as to require an 8-hour shift. So far, positions in which nursing faculty hold joint appointments have not been implemented without escalation of the number of positions and costs.

We need to plan for faculty to combine teaching, clinical practice, and research so that the faculty are not required to perform two full-time functions. For example, a program of three terms of teaching and one term of clinical practice would provide the faculty with the opportunity to build and maintain clinical background skills, identify research areas, and collect research data during clinical practice. However, this would not fully resolve the issue of how to provide students with the opportunity to observe and learn by good example from clinical experience, since services of high quality are too seldom seen in the real world.

A second possibility is to have faculty with joint appointments serve in some position in nursing service that does not require an 8-hour shift or 24-hour responsibility. These positions might be in such places as specialty outpatient clinics, inservice education, community services, or consultation might be offered on a continuing basis. These assignments would have to depend on the interest and versatility of the faculty, as well as on the needs of the nursing services organization. Consideration would have to be given to how to avoid overloading faculty if these duties are assigned in addition to their academic responsibilities, as well as how to avoid the escalating costs that result from providing services to patients/clients.

Several possibilities exist for nursing service staff to contribute to the educational efforts in the framework of the 8-hour shift arrangement. For example, appointments as preceptors or docents could be made. A *docent* has been defined by the University of Missouri, Kansas City Medical School as follows:

> A full-time physician responsible for the education of a small number of students. The *Docent* is a role model for students and serves as a guide and mentor. In a very real sense, the *Docent* serves as society's representative while he has responsibility of guiding a small group of students through the experience necessary to acquire a specified beginning clinical competence.[6]

The docent demonstrates by example how to provide comprehensive, compassionate health care.

This description would be equally applicable for highly skilled nurses who were members of a nursing services organization. Another possibility is that the nursing students could be assisted by the nurses in an agency to maintain high performance standards. The students could use these nurses as resource persons and the faculty might also request some formal classroom participation from them. The third possibility is the joint appointment whereby persons would be paid from two budgets with a stipulated assignment which would reflect the allocation of funds.

Certain conclusions can be made about the relationship between nursing services and nursing education.

1. Nursing has major responsibility for the care of patients/clients, including the modifications that must be made in activities of daily living and in the milieu.

2. The faculty in nursing can make important contributions to the departments of nursing services through selected assignments.

3. When nursing services personnel become involved in education or the faculty in nursing services becomes extensive, budgetary consideration becomes necessary.

4. All faculty should do research or perform nursing services in addition to their academic responsibilities. Such commitments could be formally recognized by the title of "Nurse Associate," which would give the faculty member research and practice privileges within the nursing services organization.

5. All health service organizations should provide a learning environment for educating health professionals as a by-product of their health services. These facilities should be created to serve the patient needs and require a basic financial outlay which will not be drastically changed by use in the preparation of professionals, since major physical expansion and use of additional resources will not usually be required.

6. The learning environment should provide health workers with the opportunity to learn and to work in association and collaboration with other professionals, and it should not be necessary to purchase this opportunity from professionals or to make payments to the various services for the placement of students in these areas.

7. Students should have an opportunity to observe and participate as various health professionals work together to provide services to individuals and families.

8. The department of nursing services in health agencies should provide learning experiences for nursing students within

all of its units, contingent on agreements with academic units in nursing.

9. The allocation of space for the teaching activities may present a problem which has to be resolved by the agency and the academic unit in nursing.

The aim should be to establish a community of scholars not unlike the community of scholars in other disciplines, but with recognition of the special needs of professional practice, as is so in medical education and other health fields.

Budgetary provisions for teachers must be adequate to ensure proper instruction of both graduate and undergraduate students. It may be necessary to seek additional funds from within and outside the university. The faculty will want to explore grants provided by the state and federal governments, as well as private foundations. Funds for teaching improvement projects and for traineeships and scholarships may be available from the Division of Nursing, a part of the Bureau of Health Manpower in the Health Resources Administration, and from such sources as the National Institute of Mental Health and Drug Abuse.

Students

In a survey of the qualities important in good nursing care of geriatric patients, Nyapadi[7] reported that patience is first and is often demanded unconsciously by old people. Other qualities reported in order of importance were observation, kindness, humor, interest, thoughtfulness, practical ability, and initiative. One writer considers maturity, "which implies a basic emotional stability which respects the humanity of all persons regardless of age or physical infirmity"[8] the primary characteristic needed by the geriatric nurse. Hodkinson lists the qualities of a good geriatric nurse:

> The ward sister in a geriatric or chronic sick hospital needs to be a good administrator, a good leader, and a home maker. She must have a wide knowledge of senescence and senility. She must know about the public health services, voluntary organizations, and all details regarding the welfare services. She must be a good teacher,

able to convey her knowledge to the patients, relatives, and all grades of staff. She must have infinite patience, never be discouraged, be tactful, sympathetic, understanding, and firm; she must be a friend to all her patients, but never identify herself with them.[9]

While not all students can realistically be expected to possess all these virtues, it would be advisable for prospective graduate students to have had some intensive experience in working with elderly people so that they may evaluate their own interests in, as well as aptitudes for, this specialized area of nursing. Graduate faculty can evaluate interest and, to some degree, aptitude, by requesting an autobiographical statement and outline of career goals as a part of the admissions application.

The aim of graduate education should be to provide an environment in which research and other kinds of scholarly efforts can be promoted, and in which graduate students may learn research and/or university teaching in a productive preceptor/mentor relationship. Even if traineeships, and federal funding for nursing programs are available, the budgeting of funds for teaching assistants is important, not only to provide needed financial support, but also to provide the appropriate educational experiences for graduate students in nursing. We have long perpetuated a situation in which nursing faculty did not have research assistants or graduate assistants as other faculty do. Continuation of this situation, we believe, results in very limited research productivity in nursing.

When there are no graduate assistantships available or when all students are supported on fellowships or traineeships, faculty may wish to implement a *professional socialization* requirement. The student would choose a preceptor for an experience in teaching, research, clinical practice, or community service. Upon enrollment in the program, the student would consult the list of faculty research and special interests and make an appointment to discuss with a preceptor career goals in relation to the experiences the preceptor may be able to offer. An outline of the proposed experience would be developed. As soon as the student has found a preceptor with whom to satisfy the professional socialization requirement, the professor-in-charge of the graduate program would be given the completed notice of intent to be kept on file. Such a notice will constitute a valid assignment. If the preceptor relationship becomes infeasible, the matter would be discussed with the professor-in-charge of the graduate program and the student would consult the faculty interest list in order to arrange for another preceptor. It is suggested that the student spend approximately five hours a week for three terms in this preceptor relationship. Adjustments may be made from term to term but should average out to this amount of time at the end of three terms. The preceptor should be able to provide professional recommendations for the students when they are ready to seek positions. Students who hold graduate assistantships for three terms would have met the requirements for the professional socialization apprenticeships. Statements of evaluation from the preceptor would be filed in the student's record.

The purpose of professional socialization is to provide for the development of a commitment to a particular specialization. Students would attend meetings of nursing organizations and other appropriate associations, such as the Gerontological Society, and may be provided experiences in presenting papers and publishing as well as experiences participating in various community services with guidance and support from faculty. An alternative to this approach might be a three- to four-month preceptorship at the end of the program to provide real-life career experiences.

According to Felton,[10] the time for giving a professional identity that is believable to oneself and others and sustainable is during the period of graduate education. Felton believes that graduate education should develop professional conduct, which includes superior technical performance and independent functioning. However, we believe the formation of a nurse's professional identity begins in the undergraduate program, should continue in graduate school, and be further developed from nursing experience. Development of professional identity is a lifelong process.

Students need shared experiences with faculty. More than a stipulated number of courses and credit hours is necessary to forge a professional identity. Too often, faculty and students do not give professional socialization serious consideration. And too often this responsibility is placed on the employing organization or agency, which has neither the resources nor expertise to fulfill it. Then the profession as a whole suffers from loss of potential leaders and low levels of professional commitment.

Admission Requirements

The admission requirements of the graduate school should be adhered to, and in addition, applicants should be graduates of a National League for Nursing accredited baccalaureate program.* They may be required to take the Graduate Record Examination or some similar examination, and to submit letters of recommendation attesting to their professional competence at the staff nurse level and their scholarship ability. Upon admission to the graduate program, each student should be assigned to an advisor or an advisory committee for counseling and program supervision, including thesis for the M.S. degree or paper for the M.N. degree. Comprehensive final examinations may be required in the content areas of the program. These should be designed to measure the achievement of the behavioral objectives of the program.

A Framework for Graduate Programs

In America a formal educational framework for geriatric or gerontological nursing practice has not yet been established. The American Nurses' Association did not recognize geriatric nursing as a nursing specialty until 1966. What is available is a definition of geriatric nursing practice and a set of standards which were first developed in 1970 by the Committee on Standards for Geriatric Nursing Practice[11] and revised in 1976[12]; and *Guidelines for Short-term Continuing Education Programs Preparing the Geriatric Nurse Practitioner.*[13] Some inferences about the basic knowledge needed for gerontic nursing practice may be drawn from the

*Graduates from nonaccredited undergraduate programs in nursing and those with other bachelor degrees should be evaluated to determine individual deficiencies and so that a program may be designed to meet these deficiencies before or concurrently with graduate study.

certification process. In addition, inferences for education may also be drawn from the Secretary's (of Health, Education and Welfare) Committee to Study Extended Roles for Nurses.[14]

In the British literature, one of the first frameworks, suggested by Norton,[15] advocated the inclusion of geriatric nursing in the general nurse training.

As could be expected, most of the articles about education for geriatric nursing are concerned with basic preparation.* We could locate no published articles about graduate education for the nursing care of the elderly until the January–February, 1977, issue of the *Journal of Gerontological Nursing*. Thus, with little literature available on graduate education, we were fortunate to have access to the experiences of the project director and project staff in nursing education, geriatrics, and gerontology at the Pennsylvania State University. In addition, a graduate program in Adult Health and Aging for the preparation of health nursing specialists begun at the University (the first students were admitted in 1973) provided some ideas and experiences that were useful in writing this chapter.

The following assumptions represent an attempt to provide guidelines for the structure of graduate education for the nursing care of the elderly.

Assumption: Graduate level preparation in nursing is built on baccalaureate level preparation in nursing.

1. Students will have common knowledge and skills in the nursing care of the elderly at a beginning professional level
2. Students will have basic knowledge of the aging process, stages of development, and the problems and factors that affect the aging population
3. Basic knowledge and skills will be maintained and used in specialized nursing practice
4. Graduate students can make up for basic deficiencies through undergraduate-level courses and experiences

*The articles that consider education at this level—for aides and practical nurses—and those that consider continuing education are discussed in chapters 4, 5, and 9. Several articles about the role of the nurse practitioner in the nursing care of the elderly are discussed in chapter 8.

Assumption: Graduate-level preparation includes specialization in areas of nursing practice.

    1. Suitable areas include health nursing; primary care; long-term care. (Acute and intensive care are not included because it has not been demonstrated that older patients need special acute and intensive care)
    2. Many elements in the nursing care of the elderly are common to health nursing, primary care, and long-term care
    3. Preparation for teaching and administration in the nursing care of the elderly will require additional courses, in addition to specialization in nursing practice

Assumption: Graduate-level preparation requires graduate courses in aging from a multidisciplinary perspective.

    1. Students will have access to courses offered in other university departments
    2. The program will be structured so as to require graduate study of the aging processes
    3. There will be collaboration between nursing faculty and other university faculty who have research interests or program interests in aging

Assumption: A variety of clinical and social services and facilities will be available for student field and practicum experiences

    1. Field experiences and experiences with the elderly will be a required component of most courses
    2. Formal arrangements will be made between faculty and agencies for student experiences
    3. The team concept and professional interdependence as well as independence will be taught through field and practicum experiences

Assumption: Training for research and the use of research funding will be incorporated throughout the period of graduate study.

1. There will be formal research methodology courses available in nursing and in other disciplines applicable to nursing
2. There need not be specific research courses developed for students specializing in the nursing care of the elderly. Rather, in all of the courses taken, students should be encouraged to use nursing data on the elderly and to work on problems that have significant implications for nursing the elderly
3. Some faculty will be engaged in research and will indicate a willingness to work with students
4. A thesis or clinical paper will be required to demonstrate the student's competence

Assumption: Study of professional issues and ethics will be incorporated in the graduate programs.

1. Formal courses will be offered in nursing or in other units such as philosophy and/or medicine which consider ethics, current issues, and problems in health care delivery
2. By guidance, advising, and example, faculty will assist in the professional socialization of students

Assumption: Preparation for beginning-level teaching positions will be based on specialization in clinical nursing.

1. Students preparing for careers in teaching will also have specialization in health nursing, primary care, or long-term care
2. The graduate courses in curriculum and instruction will usually be offered by the academic unit in education
3. Practicum experiences in teaching will be offered in the content areas of nursing care of the elderly
4. Special-topic and seminar courses in teaching may be offered

Assumption: Preparation for administration of nursing services in long-term care will be based on nursing specialization in long-term care.

1. Students preparing for careers in administration in long-term care facilities will also have specialization in long-term care nursing
2. The graduate courses in administration will usually be offered by the academic unit in business administration
3. Practicum experiences in administration will be offered in long-term care facilities
4. Special-topic and seminar courses in administration may be offered

Assumption: Graduates will require life-long learning opportunities through additional formal education, continuing education, independent study, and other methods

1. The graduate programs should provide a sound foundation on which additional preparation can occur and which will support lifelong learning
2. Programs should be realistic in length and appropriate to the degree to be earned rather than attempt to incorporate all that is known in a specialized area
3. The faculty should assume some responsibility for providing for lifelong learning opportunities

Assumption: Graduates of these programs of study should be encouraged to develop strong professional identities.

1. Students should become aware of the professional associations in nursing and gerontology, and should be encouraged to become members and to attend professional meetings
2. Students should become aware of public and voluntary agencies and organizations that are concerned with the welfare of the elderly, and should be encouraged to participate in them
3. Students should be encouraged to seek ANA certification in their special areas
4. Students should be encouraged to publish in appropriate professional journals

Expected Competencies at the Master's Level for Nurses Specializing in Health Nursing

Health nursing emphasizes the promotion of health and healthy development, using teaching, advising, counseling, and demonstration techniques, and encompasses primary, secondary, and tertiary prevention with the aged. It includes preparation for evaluating health; maintaining health surveillance of the aged in protective living settings and in group health programs; and identifying the need for assistance in planning and implementing changes in life style, health habits, and living and social arrangements affecting health.

Nurses prepared at the Master's level with an option in health nursing must be able to demonstrate:

1. Knowledge and skill in assessing the health of individuals and families
2. Skill in assessing community resources and needs for health care and assisting clients to use available resources
3. Knowledge and skill in providing immunization and screening for early detection of disease, such as eye disease, diabetes, and cancer
4. Skill in helping patients develop coping and compensatory mechanisms, moral codes, and philosopy adequate to meet stresses and crises of living, through counseling and advising
5. Skill in implementing rehabilitation and early treatment prescribed by the physician to stop the progress of disease and prevent complications
6. Knowledge and skill in helping patients prevent further illness as a result of sequelae from disease
7. Knowledge and skill in helping patients prevent accidents and the spread of infection
8. Knowledge and skill in health teaching, promoting health and preventing diseases and disabilities, and maintaining vigor for individuals, families, and groups
9. Skill in making appropriate referrals for continuity of

patient and health care and in coordinating resources and services for a particular person

10. Knowledge and skill in conducting nurse clinics for continuing care of selected patients
11. Skill in evaluating the results of health nursing activities and client outcomes.

Expected Competencies at the Master's Level for Nurses Specializing in Primary Care

Primary Care is defined as (a) a person's first contact in any given episode of illness with the health care system that leads to a decision of what must be done to resolve his problem; and (b) the responsibility for the continuum of care—that is maintenance of health, evaluation and management of symptoms, and appropriate referrals.[16]

Nurses prepared at the master's level with an option in primary care must be able to demonstrate:

1. Knowledge and skill in case finding, medical, and social agency referral
2. Skill in health surveillance of patients discharged with therapeutic regimens, homebound invalids, and persons in rest and nursing homes
3. Skill in identifying the need for, and help in, planning and implementing changes in living arrangements
4. Knowledge and skill in evaluating deviations from normality
5. Knowledge and skill in assessing the responses of patients to illness and their compliance with treatment
6. Skill in performing selected diagnostic procedures, e.g., laboratory tests, wound care
7. Skill in screening patients having problems requiring differential medical diagnosis and medical therapy
8. Skill in eliciting and recording a health history
9. Knowledge and skill in making diagnoses, choosing, initiating, and modifying selected therapies
10. Skill in using assessments to plan nursing care

11. Knowledge and skill in prescribing modifications needed by patients in diet, exercise, relief from pain, and adaptation to handicaps or impairments
12. Skill in the managing care for selected patients within protocols mutually agreed upon by nursing and medical personnel
13. Skill in consulting and collaborating with physicians, other health professionals, and the public in planning, coordinating, and instituting health care programs
14. Knowledge and skill in providing appropriate emergency treatment for cardiac arrest, shock, or hemorrhage
15. Skill in providing appropriate information to the patient and his family about a diagnosis or plan of therapy
16. Skill in evaluating nursing care and client/patient outcomes.

Many of the items on this list were adapted from those presented by the Secretary's Committee to Study Extended Roles for Nurses.[17] Some additions have been added.

Expected Competencies at the Master's Level for
Nurses Specializing in Long-term Care

According to Anderson, Cooley, and Sparrow:

Long-term care consists of those services designed to provide symptomatic treatment, maintenance,and rehabilitative services for patients in all age groups in a variety of health care settings. The emphasis here is on the care required by the elderly.[18]

It should include preparation for maintaining chronically ill patients, such as those in nursing homes or other institutions for long-term care, in a stable state; assessing changes in conditions; planning nursing care; preventing complications; instituting rehabilitative measures; and consulting with the physician as conditions necessitating changes in the medically prescribed therapeutic regimes change. It should also provide appropriate conditions for the dying patient when therapeutic intervention is not possible.

Nurses prepared at the Master's level with an option in long-term care must be able to demonstrate:

1. Skill in securing and maintaining a health history
2. Skill in assessing physical and psychological states
3. Skill in assisting patient and family to identify needed resources
4. Skill in making necessary changes in a treatment plan
5. Knowledge and skill in providing continuous health guidance until all practical rehabilitation of patient has been achieved, or supportive care as needed until death
6. Skill in instituting immediate lifesaving measures in the absence of a physician
7. Knowledge and skill in giving treatments, rehabilitative exercises, and medications as prescribed by the physician
8. Knowledge and skill in teaching the patient, or family members, or other caretakers to give medication or treatments, taking cultural, psychological, and socioeconomic factors in consideration
9. Skill in continual observation and recording to indicate change in patient's condition
10. Knowledge and skill in instituting and maintaining therapeutic environments
11. Within the protocols mutually agreed upon by medical and nursing staff, knowledge and skill in: making adjustments in medication; requesting and interpreting laboratory tests; making judgments about the use of accepted pharmaceutical agents as standard treatment in diagnosed conditions; assuming primary responsibility for determining possible alternatives for care settings and for initiating referrals
12. Knowledge and skill in conducting nurse clinics for continuing care of selected patients
13. Knowledge and skill in conducting community clinics for case finding and screening for health problems
14. Knowledge and skill in assessing community needs in long-term care and participating in the development of resources to meet them
15. Willingness to assume responsibility for the environment as it affects quality and effectiveness of care
16. Skill in evaluating nursing care and patient outcomes

Graduate Education 111

17. Skill in coordinating health and community services for the benefit of particular clients

Many of the items on this list were adapted from those presented by the Secretary's Committee to Study Extended Roles for Nurses.[19] Some additions have been made.

Expected Competencies at the Master's Level for the Nurse Administrator of Long-term Care Facilities

The nurse should be able to demonstrate the following, in addition to the general competencies outlined for long-term care:

1. Knowledge and understanding of the basic principles and theories underlying clinical practice
2. Knowledge, techniques, and skill needed for effective leadership and management in health care settings
3. Knowledge and skill in formulating and implementing goals and budgetary procedures and methods of professional accountability
4. Knowledge and skill in handling relations between the client and health care personnel
5. Understanding and skill in making administrative decisions and using research findings
6. Knowledge and skill in establishing therapeutic and prosthetic environments; willingness to assume responsibility for the environment as it affects quality and effectiveness of care
7. Skill in evaluating nursing care and patient outcomes
8. Skill in communicating with other administrators, governing bodies, and the public

Expected Competencies at the Master's Level for the Nurse Educator

The nurse should be able to demonstrate the following competencies in addition to those outlined for health nursing, primary care, and long-term care:

1. Knowledge of curriculum theory and development and skills necessary to establish teaching-learning environments
2. Knowledge and skills necessary to teach and evaluate teaching
3. Skill in designing modular and course materials for use in teaching
4. Knowledge of academic settings, their politics, and acceptable role behaviors

Curriculum Framework for Doctoral Programs with a Minor in Nursing

Assumption:

Five to ten nurses with Ph.Ds, all of whom are vigorous, some of whom are nationally visible, several of whom have research under way and whose research is being quoted by other investigators, more than constitute a critical mass for a Ph.D. in nursing that would be as robust as fully half the so-called hard Ph.D. degrees being offered by all disciplines in this country.[20]

1. Faculty with senior membership in the graduate school may serve as chairmen or members of doctoral and dissertation committees
2. Faculty with associate membership in the graduate school may serve as members of doctoral and dissertation committees

Assumption: The Doctor of Philosophy is conferred in recognition of high attainment and productive scholarship in some special field of learning, as evidenced by the satisfactory completion of a prescribed period of study and investigation; the preparation of a thesis involving independent research; and the successful passing of examinations covering both the special subject and the general field of learning in which this subject forms a part

1. The core knowledge base for a nurse gerontologist should consist of advanced biology, physiology, human

development, psychology, and social gerontology, with specialized professional preparation in nursing
2. The advanced professional preparation in nursing may be obtained in the graduate-level nursing courses (offered to students enrolled for the Master's degree) and in seminar courses
3. The nurse preparing for a career in gerontology and/or geriatrics may select a major program for study according to career goals from a variety of departments in the university, including the following:
   a. academic curriculum and instruction
   b. anthropology
   c. biology
   d. community systems planning and development
   e. counselor education
   f. educational psychology
   g. human development and family studies
   h. physiology
   i. political science
   j. psychology
   k. sociology
4. Interdisciplinary majors involving two or more departments in a college or intercollege majors involving two or more colleges may be arranged with the approval of the dean of the graduate school. These programs are offered under the supervision of appropriate interdepartmental or intercollege committees

Assumption: The ability to do independent research and competence in scholarly exposition must be demonstrated by the preparation of a dissertation on some topic related to the major area and which represents a significant contribution to knowledge.

1. The academic unit in nursing should develop a vigorous research climate in gerontology and gerontic nursing, as training for research is best accomplished in an apprenticeship-preceptor or scientist-mentor relationship
2. Seminars on research and activities should be developed

and offered, including discussions of theoretical formulations, methodologies, and findings. These should be interdisciplinary in nature.
3. Research and training grants should be sought for the support of studies and programs in aging, gerontology, and gerontic nursing

Expected Competencies at the Doctoral Level

The nurse prepared at the doctoral level should be able to demonstrate:

1. Specialized knowledge of biology, physiology, human development, psychology, social gerontology, and of the interactions between health and aging processes of the middle-aged and aged
2. Knowledge of current developments, controversies, issues, theories, and research
3. Updating and expansion of knowledge base, as evidenced by participation in professional symposia and colloquies
4. Knowledge and skill in research methodology
5. Knowledge and skill in the use of statistical procedures
6. Knowledge and skill in proposal writing for research and training grants
7. Skill in independent research and scholarly exposition, as demonstrated by the preparation of an original dissertation

Examples of a Graduate Program and Graduate Courses

The following examples of a graduate program and graduate courses illustrate some of the concepts discussed in this chapter. The graduate program is a program for specialization in Health Nursing with a clinical option in Adult Health and Aging developed for The Pennsylvania State University in 1972. Such program descriptions may be useful for advising students about the nature of the program and may serve as a guide in academic planning. It must be realized that programs will be changed from time to time according to the faculty and their interpretations of the nursing needs of the elderly, the research findings, and student and consumer response. Illustrations of possible M.S. and M.N. programs are shown below (the understanding is that most students will take more than the minimum requirements).

Sample M.N. and M.S. Degrees in Nursing Curricula

Requirements	Sample M.N. Degree (Minimum Credits=30)	Sample M.S. Degree (Minimum Credits=40)
Clinical Process Courses	10 credits	6 credits
Nursing and Health Care Courses	6 credits	6 credits
Supporting Science Courses	3 credits	4 credits
Methods of Clinical Research	3 credits	6 credits
Electives for Support of Career Goal	6 credits	12 credits
Individual Study for Clinical Paper/Thesis	2 credits	6 credits
Comprehensive Exam	Required	Required

These M.S. and M.N. degrees differ mainly in terms of the kinds of research training offered, the proportion of science and nursing process courses offered, and the inclusion of preparation for teaching or administration in the M.S. degree. Ideally, the M.S. thesis should differ clearly from the clinical paper required for the M.N. degree. The thesis should test hypotheses on the relationship between two or more variables. The clinical paper should focus on description and evaluation of nursing practice.

A Graduate Program with a Specialization in
Health Nursing and a Clinical Option in
Adult Health and Aging

1. Purpose: To prepare registered nurses for expanded roles in promoting optimum health for adults and the aged.
   a. increase knowledge of the physical, social, and behavioral sciences related to health and the aging process
   b. increase knowledge of research methods appropriate to the solution of nursing problems encountered in the promotion of health for adults and the aging
   c. increase ability to perform and evaluate methods appropriate to the promotion of health for adults and the aging, i.e., counseling, advising, demonstrating, and teaching methods
   d. increase ability to work with other professionals and the public in the development and evaluation of health resources and services
   e. increase ability to analyze and cope with problems and issues in the provision of health promotion services
2. Title of practitioner: Adult Health and Aging Specialist
3. Target population: Middle-aged and aged; more specifically, those persons over 50 years of age.
4. Bases of operation or context—practicum sites
   a. group health plans—organizations
   b. neighborhood health clinics
   c. health maintenance organizations
   d. retirement homes
   e. residential facilities for the aged
   f. senior centers and clubs
   g. public health agencies
5. Functions
   a. assess and evaluate health status using history taking and selected screening methods to evaluate deviations from normal
   b. refer to medical and social agencies
   c. maintain health surveillance of the aged in protective living settings and in group health programs

d. identify the need for assistance in the planning and implementation of changes in life style, health habits, and living and social arrangements affecting the health of individuals
e. counsel and advise individuals and families and provide self-education resources
f. conduct group teaching, discussions, and demonstrations
g. consult and collaborate with physicians, other health professionals, and the public in planning and instituting health care programs
6. Major concepts guiding practice
   a. the physical, psychological, and social processes of aging and interaction with health status
   b. the societal, socioeconomic, and political aspects of aging as these affect social and health programs and community resources
   c. the relations between people and the environment, as these relate to health and aging
   d. stress, adaptation, and health in relation to aging
   e. relation between the aged and their families, with emphasis on independency and dependency as a consequence of socialization
   f. behavioral change and therapeutic intervention
   g. principles and guides for adult education
7. Model Curriculum—M.S. Adult Health and Aging—Teaching
   a. Practicums
      1. Clinical Process in Health Care and Nursing—Health Nursing
   b. Principles and practices
      1. Physical Assessment
      2. Psychosocial Assessment
   c. Supporting science courses
      1. Adulthood
      2. Seminar in Adult Development and Aging
      3. Medication Management
   d. Clinical study and research
      1. Statistical Methods I
      2. Design and Analysis of Clinical Studies

3. Thesis
e. Career goal of administration
   1. Clinical Process in Health Care and Nursing—Clinical Teaching
   2. The Nurse Educator
   3. Theories of Learning
   4. Issues in Nursing and Health Care
8. Nursing courses
   a. Issues in Nursing and Health Care
   b. Design and Analysis of Clinical Studies in Nursing
   c. The Nurse Administrator
   d. The Nurse Educator
   e. Basic Principles of Physical Assessment
   f. Basic Principles of Psychosocial Assessment
   g. Medication Management
   h. Clinical Process in Health Care and Nursing
   i. Individual Studies in Nursing Health
   j. Special Topics in Nursing and Health
   k. Colloquium in Health Care and Nursing
   l. Thesis
9. Suggested courses in other disciplines
   a. Health Planning and Administration Epidemiologic Basis for Planning
   b. H.P.A. Economic Analysis and Health
   c. Individual and Family Studies Resolving Individual and Family Problems
   d. I.F.S. Adulthood
   e. I.F.S. Developmental Theory
   f. I.F.S. Seminar in Adult Development and Aging
   g. Human Development Research
   h. Community System Planning and Development Health Care Organization
10. Comprehensive examination

M.S. Degree	Percentage of Exam	M.N. Degree	Percentage of Exam
Nursing Process and Theory	25	Nursing Process Nursing Theory	30 40

Supporting		Clinical Studies	20
Sciences	20	General	
Research	20	Professional Area	10
General			
Professional Area	10		
Functional Area			
(Administration or			
Teaching)	25		

11. Criteria for evaluating thesis and clinical paper

   A clinical paper describes *a clinical problem* and provides *implications* or suggestions for *the improvement of nursing practice* that can be shared with other practitioners (*ANA Guidelines*).
   a. The paper is more informal than the thesis. It may:
      1. describe, interpret, or explain nursing practice in a single case in any setting
      2. present generalizations drawn from several cases of the same clinical nursing problem in one or in different settings (e.g., hospital, home)
      3. present findings of investigations and their implications for clinical nursing practice
      4. show the synthesis of knowledge and demonstrate its use in developing a plan of action in a particular clinical nursing problem and in contributing towards the formulation of nursing theory
      5. report an original investigation or critically evaluate a published work
   b. A thesis is a formal research endeavor that typically requires generation of new data.* It should:
      1. indicate the student's capacity to describe a scientific inquiry in writing
      2. evidence the student's ability to formulate and define the purpose of an investigation, study, critical analysis, or evaluation
      3. show the student's ability to acquire and analyze information

*For a discussion of criteria used to evaluate theses, see *Nursing Outlook*, (August, 1964): 60, prepared by the staff of the NLN Research Studies Service.

4. show the student's ability to draw logical conclusions
5. show the student's ability to relate findings to professional problems and practices in nursing
   c. The evidence of the student's competence comes from two sources: the faculty's report on the development of the paper or thesis, including the number of conferences necessary, the student's independence of thought and general approach to the problem; and the faculty's estimation of the finished paper or thesis.
12. Suggested research and clinical problems for study
   Studies in health nursing may be categorized broadly under the following topics:
   a. attitudes, preferences, and job satisfaction in care of the aged
   b. psychosocial techniques and approaches in the care of the aged
   c. clinical problems and protection in care of the aged
   d. health in the aging process
   e. health promotion activities—methods and efficacy
   f. correlates of health in old age
   g. self-care activities in the preservation of health, vigor, and functions in old age. (This option will require studies on health in the aging process and methods and efficacy of various health promotion activities.)
13. Employment opportunities
   a. administrators of nursing services in public health, H.M.O.s
   b. practitioner and consultant in senior centers, retirement homes, neighborhood health centers, group health plans
   c. teacher in adult health and aging—community health courses and staff development programs

A Master of Science Degree with Preparation for
Teaching Gerontic Nursing

1. Purpose
   a. provide knowledge to function as a teacher
   b. give student practice in applying learning theory

c. give student an understanding of curriculum development
d. help student design modular and course materials for use in teaching
e. give student practice in evaluation (test construction)
f. give student practice in using measurement materials
g. give student practice in using a variety of teaching methods
2. Title of practitioner: Nursing Educator
3. Bases of operation or context—practicum sites
The undergraduate program would provide the population or practicum sites for the teaching option. This would include formal classroom teaching/laboratory learning and clinical practicum areas
4. Functions
The student would learn to carry out all activities commonly associated with teaching in a nursing setting
   a. construct program goals and objectives
   b. assess student characteristics
   c. develop learning objectives
   d. derive subject content based on objectives
   e. develop pretest items
   f. select teaching/learning activities and resources
   g. evaluate achievement
5. Nursing courses
   a. The Nurse Educator
   b. Clinical Process in Health Care and Nursing—Teaching
   c. Colloquium
   d. Individual Studies
6. Suggested courses in other disciplines/colleges
   a. Instructional Design
      1. Orientation to Instructional Media
      2. Production and Utilization of Graphic Stimulus Materials
      3. Production of Educational Motion Pictures
      4. Television in Education
   b. Teaching Methodology
      1. Philosophic Basis of Education
   c. Educational Psychology

1. Statistical Interpretation of Educational Research
2. Applied Parametric and Nonparametric Statistics in Education
3. Learning Processes in Relation to Educational Practices
4. Current Topics in Educational Psychology
5. Group Processes in the Classroom
6. Contemporary Learning Models in Educational Psychology
7. Psychological Foundations for College Teaching
8. Concept Learning in the Schools
9. Theories of Learning and Instruction
10. Survey of Media Research
d. Educational Administration
 1. Organizational Supervision
 2. Theory and Practice of Educational Negotiations
e. Higher Education
 1. Higher Education in the United States
 2. College Teaching
 3. Curriculums in Higher Education
 4. Community Junior College and the Technical Institute
 5. Administration in Higher Education
 6. The History of American Higher Education
 7. Seminar in Higher Education
 8. College Students
7. Comprehensive examination
 a. The student should be able to respond verbally and in writing to questions about the teacher's role and other related behaviors of nursing educators, such as
  1. instructional design
  2. learning theory
  3. evaluative approaches
8. Criteria for evaluating thesis
 a. relevant to teaching
 b. adds to knowledge student gained during program work
 c. includes current research in the field
 d. provides student with reference material

e. is scholarly in character and follows acceptable format for presentation, e.g., the *Publication Manual* of the American Psychological Association (APA)
9. Suggested research and problems for study
  a. entering behaviors of nursing students
  b. designs for instruction in a specific content area
  c. development of instructional objective data bank
  d. effect of specific instructional pattern on student achievement
  e. individualization of nursing instruction
10. Employment opportunities
  a. baccalaureate nursing programs throughout the United States
  b. nursing educator consultant in media development companies
  c. staff development positions

Courses in the Graduate Curriculum

Graduate courses will be drawn from gerontology, nursing, gerontic nursing, and education and nursing or business administration. Electives may be taken in any number of disciplines. Each program will be tailored to the parent university and the academic unit in nursing.

The courses in gerontology might include courses such as the Biology of Aging, Psychopathology of Aging, and the Economics and Politics of Aging. Other courses may be selected depending on a student's research interests and on the interests of faculty. For example, seminars and independent or special topic courses might be offered, such as Clinical Diagnosis and Treatment of the Aged, Disease Processes and Behavior in the Aged, and Adaptations to Stress in the Aged.

Some upper-division courses may be open to both undergraduate and graduate students. These courses should emphasize activities that require interpretation and/or synthesis of information, use of concepts and principles to solve new problems, evaluation and/or critique of studies, and applications of specific methods and techniques.

Graduate courses open only to graduate students should, in addition, emphasize the evaluation of arguments; utilization of standards to evaluate papers and reports; formulation of hypotheses, theories, and experiments or projects; and the analysis of data as a basis for drawing conclusions.

Some graduate courses should meet students' needs no matter what the students' areas of specialization and options may be. Examples are: Issues in Nursing and Health Care; Design and Analysis of Clinical Studies in Nursing; Basic Principles of Physical Assessment; Basic Psychosocial Principles in Health Assessment; Medication Management; Colloquia; Individual Studies; and Special Topics.

Examples of Course Outlines

Course:
Issues in Health Care
Credit Hours:
2:2:0
Prerequisites:
None

Description:
Consideration of personal, social, political, economic, philosophical, or ethical problems/questions, and ways of confronting and resolving conflicts in professional practice.

Brief Outline:
1. Concepts of human rights
   a. the meaning of freedom, responsibility, and choice
   b. the right to health
   c. the right to healthy environments
2. Health issues associated with secondary effects of science and technology
   a. why excessive population growth is a health-related problem
   b. increase in chronic disease and disability (an aging population)
   c. nursing and health issues arising from pollution of the environment

3. Present concerns
    a. control of population growth
        1. abortion
        2. euthanasia
        3. suicide
        4. prolongation of life
    b. the right to live
        1. survival of defective children
        2. procreation of people who carry defective genes
        3. procreation of the mentally retarded
        4. the relationship between poverty and disease
    c. decisions on death
        1. who should have the use of lifesaving technologies?
        2. who should pay for the expensive lifesaving technologies?
        3. who should make the decision whether or not to use life saving technology?
4. The ethics of medical research
    a. the protection of human subjects
    b. informed consent
    c. should the patient benefit?
5. The ethics of medical and social services
    a. why should people care?
    b. how should people care?
    c. human behavior control

Evaluation:
Students will be evaluated on the basis of a major project or paper and on discussion contributions.

Course:
Design and Analysis of Clinical Studies in Nursing*
Credit Hours:
3:3:0

*This course will provide the experience in research technique to enable students to fulfill the M.N. degree requirement for a clinical paper and M.S. degree requirement for a thesis. The collection of data, analysis of results, and the writing of the report and/or thesis will be done in the course in Individual Studies in Health Care and Nursing and/or in the Thesis course.

Prerequisites:
Statistics or courses that provide fundamental knowledge of statistics

Description:
Research design for problems of developing and evaluating nursing care programs, products, methods, and procedures

Brief Outline:
1. Introduction to clinical research in nursing
    a. implications of the debate on "pure" versus "applied" research and experimental versus clinical research
    b. differences between problem solving and research in clinical work
    c. characteristics of the criteria for clinical studies
2. Goals and examples of research in clinical nursing
    a. improvement of patient care—health promotion, maintenance, restoration, and rehabilitation
    b. utilization of health and nursing manpower
    c. expansion of nursing responsibilities in the health care system
    d. enrichment of the curriculum in nursing education
    e. improving the organization of nursing services
3. The scientific method in clinical nursing research
    a. derivation and formulation of hypotheses
    b. kinds of research: descriptive, exploratory, experimental; their importance
    c. theoretical basis for determination of variables, selection of methods, and data collection techniques, and illustrations from biological and behavioral sciences
    d. sampling problems in incidence and expost facto studies
    e. protection of human subjects
4. Development of the clinical design
    a. systematic review of literature
    b. formulation of a purpose
    c. choice of method as a function of purpose
    d. description of analysis proposed
    e. presentation of proposal for critical review

Justification and Evaluation:
1. The general aims are to provide:
   a. stimulation of interest in use of the scientific method and the development of research hypotheses in relation to nursing problems through discussion, review of literature, and analysis of selected studies
   b. knowledge and understanding of the scientific method and problems in research, such as inference, causality, measurement, design, data collection techniques, analysis of data, and organization of the report
   c. knowledge of some of the simpler sociological, psychological, and biological techniques which may be useful in the study of nursing problems, with illustrations from the nursing literature
   d. experience and opportunity to develop skill in the process of developing a research design
2. The student's progress will be measured in terms of the specific objectives. At the conclusion of the course the student should be able to:
   a. abstract research studies
   b. evaluate research studies
   c. identify an area suitable for study
   d. review the literature in the area identified for study of both the theoretical constructs as well as the recent research findings
   e. present the review of the literature in a paper, using proper thesis format
   f. develop a proposal for the solution of a problem in nursing
   g. answer correctly items concerning the assigned readings on an objective-answer final examination: 85% correct items for grade of A; 75% correct items for grade of B
3. There will be no duplication of instructional efforts in other academic units.

Course:
Individual Studies in Nursing and Health

Credit Hours:
Variable credit is needed because graduate nursing students have a wide range of backgrounds and different lengths of time are required for students to develop competency. Four hours of experience per week will be required per credit granted.
Prequisites:
Permission of instructor
Description:
Creative projects include non-thesis research, under individual supervision, on topics which fall outside the scope of formal courses.
Justification:
Graduate nursing students enrolled in the Master of Nursing option will be required to complete non-thesis research.

Courses in Nursing Specializations

The advantage of having approved courses and descriptions general enough to provide for specialization and options includes the ability to modify experiences and content without having to have such modifications approved by the graduate school or faculty senate. Two such courses are illustrated here. These courses are based on courses in physical assessment and psychosocial assessment as prerequisites. The clinical-process courses also require a practicum component. Several types of clinical facilities and social agencies may be used to provide appropriate experiences. Some students may elect to work in two or more settings. This experience should be planned with each student and based on previous experiences and career goals.

Examples of Course Outlines
Course:
Clinical Process in Health Care and Nursing
Credit Hours:
3–10
Prerequisites:
Completion of advanced nursing theory courses in selected clini-

cal or functional areas, or permission of instructor. Courses in physical and psychosocial assessment.

Description:
Supervised experience to develop competence in selected clinical or functional areas of health care or nursing practice.

Brief Outline:
1. Intensive experience in the delivery of health care, specialized clinical nursing, the teaching of nursing, or nursing administration
2. Continuous interaction with members of other health professions in a collaborative role
3. Opportunity for the development and testing of health care and nursing theories
4. Opportunity to identify the unknown in health care and nursing

Justification and Evaluation:
1. Upon completion of the course the student should be able to:
   a. demonstrate knowledge and skills in specific area selected for graduate study in nursing and health care
   b. demonstrate an ability to function as a member of the health team
2. The student will be evaluated by instructor observations of the clinical situation, instructor review and evaluation of patients' records, as well as instructor evaluation of the student's oral and written analyses of certain clinical cases and situations.

Content to be included in health nursing, primary care, and long-term care is outlined below and would be offered in a course such as clinical process in health care and nursing with a practicum component.

Health Nursing
1. Health, disease, and aging interactions
   a. physical aspects
   b. psychological aspects
   c. social aspects
   d. ecological aspects

2. Health promotion
    a. primary prevention
    b. secondary prevention
    c. tertiary prevention
3. Techniques for assessment of the aged
    a. physical
    b. behavioral
    c. functional
    d. social
    e. health screening
4. Techniques applicable to health promotion in the aged
    a. diagnosis of learner needs and assessment of resources
    b. small-group techniques
    c. behavioral techniques
    d. development of teaching materials including demonstrations
    e. advising and counseling processes for the aged
    f. evaluation and research
5. Utilization of resources—medical, rehabilitation, nursing, recreational, and social
    a. interprofessional and intraprofessional activities
    b. collaboration
    c. consultation
    d. communication and resolution of conflicts
    e. community, state, and national resources
6. Philosophical and ethical issues
    a. patient's rights
    b. differences in values
    c. culture and health

Primary Care Nursing

1. Concepts of health and disease in the aging
    a. physical function and pathology of common diseases
    b. psychological health and mental disease
    c. functional disabilities
    d. application of assessment methods, including laboratory findings

2. Management of common diseases and disorders affecting the aged
   a. development of protocols
   b. drug management or monitoring
   c. referral and consultation
   d. crisis management and emergency care
   e. continuity of care
   f. teaching clients and family
3. Records and evaluation
   a. history-taking and observation
   b. systems of recording and reporting
   c. peer evaluation and relationships
   d. quality assurance
4. Management of time and costs
   a. office and clinic practices
   b. use of resources
   c. cost of accountability
   d. third-party payments

Long-term Care Nursing
1. Nursing in long-term care
   a. assessment of functional states, disabilities, and disease processes
   b. planning short- and long-range goals
   c. implementing the plan of care
   d. monitoring and evaluating progress
   e. using resources for maintaining functions, rehabilitation and comfort, as well as for prevention of complications.
2. Development of therapeutic milieu
   a. therapeutic and nontherapeutic effects
   b. physical components
   c. social and psychological components
   d. activities of daily living
   e. therapeutic regimen
3. Protection
   a. iatrogenic complications
   b. safety
   c. legal aspects

4. Use of auxiliary personnel
   a. in-service education and continuing education
   b. supervision
   c. stereotypes and interests of personnel in working with older people
5. Clinical problems and therapeutic advances
   a. nursing
   b. medicine
   c. issues and trends
   d. standards and types of care
6. Specific nursing care problems and research
   a. food and nutrition
   b. personal hygiene
      1. skin care
      2. mouth care
      3. dress
   c. elimination
      1. incontinence
      2. constipation
   d. behavioral disturbances
      1. confusion
      2. social withdrawal
      3. irritabiiity
      4. assaultive behavior
      5. self-mutilation and suicide
   e. sleep loss and insomnia
   f. accident prevention
   g. dying, death, and bereavement
7. Special medical problems
   a. iatrogenic disorders
   b. pneumonia
   c. cardiac decompensation
   d. diabetes control
   e. alcoholism
   f. cancer
   g. pulmonary disease
   h. malnutrition
   i. depression and other mental disorders

j. arthritis
k. fractures of hip
l. cataracts and glaucoma

The Seminar

The seminar is indispensible in graduate education that trains for clinical study and research. In the seminar students will have an opportunity to express their ideas and obtain feedback from professors and fellow students. The professors also make their contributions and receive feedback from students in a way that promotes and stimulates the intellectual development of students and teachers. Research projects may be undertaken jointly by members of the seminar under the leadership of the professor, or students may present results of their thesis or independent study effort. In any event, instruction and training regarding the nature of research, methodology, techniques, tools, and bibliographic sources should be included in the seminar.

An attempt should be made to distinguish the seminar from courses dealing with the practical aspects of nursing knowledge, such as the attainment of advanced clinical skills. A course considering specialized practice and the knowledge underlying this practice in nursing and health care should include nursing imperatives generally, and specifically the rules for the effective and moral performance of nursing. The emphasis in seminar should be on theory in the context of systematic description and explanation and verification by use of scientific methods.

Examples of Course Outlines

An outline for a seminar in nursing gerontology is offered below. It would be appropriate for students in health nursing, primary care, and long-term care.

Course:
Seminar in Nursing Gerontology
Credit Hours:
3

Prerequisites:
Completion of ¾ of Master's program
Placement of Course:
Master's, post Master's
Description:
Gerontological research findings applied to complex nursing problems in maintenance of health and maximum functioning in the aged.
Brief Outline:
1. The specific objectives are to assist the student to obtain increased knowledge of:
    a. the nature and purpose of research in gerontology
    b. the methodology and techniques of research in gerontology
    c. the tools and sources for research in gerontology
    d. the implications and/or applications of research findings for nursing practice

Evaluation:
The members of the seminar will report on their theses or on individual research projects. Discussion should be free, but well organized, and should provide opportunity for informal contact and exchange of views between faculty and students. Students will be evaluated on oral performance and written reports.

Course:
Seminar in Nursing and Health Care
Credit Hours:
2–9
Prerequisites:
Graduate nursing majors, other majors who have received permission; those who have taken courses in statistics and research methodology.
Description:
Seminar in acute and intensive, long-term or health care, nursing administration, or nursing education
Brief Outline:
1. foundations for development of clinical, administrative, or educational knowledge, skills, and attitudes in nursing

a. functions
   b. influences of societal and cultural values
   c. influence of opinions and concepts advanced by specialists in disease and health
   d. philosophical influences
   e. theories and models—clinical, administrative, or educational
2. processes and principles that facilitate development of clinical, administrative, or educational practices in nursing
   a. identification of goals
   b. identification of processes
   c. assessment of methods to facilitate processes
3. activation of clinical, administrative, or educational research methodology
   a. utilization of people
   b. use of current research and knowledge
   c. interpretation of plan
   d. initiation and adaptation of changes in the plan
4. evaluation of performance/outcome/result—clinical, administrative, or educational
   a. methods of evaluation
   b. interrelationships of evaluation, processes, and plans
5. application of clinical, administrative, or educational findings for nursing (student project)
6. identification by learner for clinical practitioner, administrator, or educator, of strengths and limitations of findings and of own ability to
   a. analyze
   b. synthesize
   c. implement
   d. evaluate

Justification:
The design of the seminars permits the graduate student to specify an emphasis in research on clinical, administrative, or educational functions. The graduate learner develops skills in analysis, synthesis, and application of theory and research from nursing and related areas. These effective methods of bringing together rational planning and human orientation are what graduate education is all about.

The course should build on the student's knowledge of nursing practice, the research process, and biological, societal, and psychological aspects of aging.

Objectives are implemented through student reports on their individual research projects, open but organized discussion, and informal contact and exchange of views between faculty and students.

Presentation of a discussion in seminar and a written paper are used to determine the student's final grade. This paper may be developed around any of the topics covered in the seminar or in any area of social gerontology or gerontic nursing. Each student is expected to make an oral presentation. For a grade of A, the student shall present an inquiry using original data gathered by the student in addition to library data. For a grade of B, the student shall present an inquiry using library data. However, the quality of the student's report will provide the basis for the final grade.

The following is a list of possible seminar topics:

Interaction of Health Status and Aging Processes
Problems in Practitioner Education
Nursing Assessments, Observations, Recordings
Organization and Management of Nursing Unit Milieu/ Evaluation of Home Milieu
Social Interaction and Care of the Older Patient/Psychosocial Nursing
Clinical Problems and Therapeutic Advances/Nursing and Medicine
Health Promotion Techniques in Aging Population Groups
Nursing Methods in Gerontic Nursing

Evaluation of Graduate Programs

Evaluation of graduate programs may be conducted in a number of ways. Most nursing programs will be accredited by the National League for Nursing. NLN accreditation indicates to the public that a program has met the NLN's stated criteria. In addition, most graduate schools have established systematic evaluation plans. This program review may consist of a self-assessment by the faculty in nursing and an outside review by a committee appointed by the graduate school. In some instances, a person outside the university may be used as a part of the review committee. The program review will usually include a description of the program, the administration, resources, instructional program, faculty, and graduates of the program. Questionnaire forms should be provided for evaluation of the program by faculty, students, graduates, and by others, intrauniversity as well as inter-university. Recommendations from the faculty making the report may be included.

The faculty will want to perform a systematic review and evaluation of the graduate program at intervals. Suggested topics to consider are:

1. The philosophy of the program
2. The relations between the philosophy and program objectives
3. The relations between the objectives for each emphasis in the program, and for the two degrees, to the behavioral objectives
4. The courses and their relations to the program objectives
5. Development or modification of a questionnaire to evaluate the educational process, the effectiveness of the faculty, and the relevance of the program to the students

Reviews should consider continuing education-community services, including the university services in most institutions. Reviews may be performed by a faculty committee. All faculty should be advised to obtain evaluations on each course taught. In this way, students have an opportunity to evaluate the courses offered in the graduate program.

The graduate school may also conduct routine, random sampling evaluations of all theses produced. Theses can be selected for review by appointed committees, and a confidential report made. The format used for the review of graduate theses by The

Pennsylvania State University includes the following questions. Each reviewer is requested to rate and provide a critical evaluation of the thesis work.

1. Is the title appropriate and concise?
2. Is the problem stated plainly?
3. Is the plan of research clear?
4. Is the thesis well and concisely written?
5. Does it seem to you to be scholarly research?
6. Is the depth of treatment appropriate?
7. Is it clear which is author's work and which is that of others?
8. Is the methodology adequate for the problem? Is sample sufficient in size and meaning?
9. Do results follow from research? Are they meaningful?
10. If a doctoral thesis, is the abstract satisfactory?

The nursing program may adapt a similar form for the evaluation of each thesis and clinical paper to be done by a departmental committee. These evaluations can then be compiled in the nursing unit.

The purpose of the discussion in chapter 7 has been to identify aspects of the administration and organization of graduate programs in gerontic nursing that are pertinent to the total milieu in which the student is educated. We believe this educational process should consist of more than learning gerontic nursing content. In addition to other courses in nursing and in other disciplines, the faculty and their relations with students, agency personnel, and professional, university and community activities all influence what a student learns. The interests, aptitudes, motivation, and experiences of students, too, have a part in the teaching-learning situation, as do the interplay between faculty and students, and the physical, social, and psychological components of the learning environment.

8
Preparing the Geriatric Nurse Practitioner

In 1948 Esther Lucille Brown suggested the need for clinical specialization in nursing, in addition to teaching, supervision, administration, and public health nursing.[1] She proposed two distinct but interrelated functions as appropriate for the clinical nurse to perform: to act as the physician's assistant in performing complex technical procedures and treatments; and to be responsible for observing patients and providing care for long periods of time without specific directions from physicians.

Twenty years later, in 1968, Silver and his coworkers reported on a four-month pediatric nurse practitioner program designed to expand the role of the nurse in order to provide increased health care for children.[2]

The next events that probably contributed to the implementation of the nurse practitioner concept were the development of the physician's assistant program at Duke University[3] and the Medex program at the University of Washington.[4] These programs were developed because it was believed that there were too few well trained health care workers to meet the demands of consumers. The medical profession was aware it was not meeting these demands. Problems in the health care system were being publicized widely. So was the need to make better use of available physicians. Preparation of a new member of the health team was viewed as a way of conserving the costly talents of the physician and making health care available in underserved areas. These programs were designed primarily to offer career opportunities to medical corpsmen discharged from the military services. Perhaps the most forceful stimulus, however, was the American Medical Association's proposal in 1970 that nurses specially trained in the fee-for-service practice of medicine supplement the criticial shortage of physicians.[5] Following this announcement, in 1970, the National Center for Health Services and Research and Development, which had been created in 1968 to conduct research related to the improvement of health services, issued a position statement on medicine and nursing in the 1970s.[6] This statement enumerated the benefits to be gained from the expansion of the role of the nurse:

1. physicians can expand their responsibilities in planning and managing programs for comprehensive care
2. physicians can concentrate on matters demanding their specialized skills
3. more services and more time and attention can be given to patients by using nurses associated with physicians
4. physicians can have more time to participate in continuing education, thereby maintaining their proficiency
5. increased status for nurses
6. increased potential to provide home care

The decision to help untangle the manpower problems resulted in a series of specially designed projects related to physician-extender personnel; PRIMEX (family nurse practitioner) and MEDEX were among those early programs.

Clarifying Terminology

The term "nurse practitioner" has recently come into common usage, although it has different meanings, and many titles are used for nurses in this role. Educational programs for the preparation of these nurses vary in sponsorship, length, and content. The problem of terminology is further complicated because any practicing nurse may be called a nurse practitioner or practitioner. In 1974, the Congress for Nursing Practice of the American Nurses' Association attempted to clarify several terms used to describe roles in nursing.[7] Practitioners of professional nursing were described as registered nurses who provide direct nursing care to people. Nurse practitioners were described as having advanced skills in assessing physical and psychosocial health-illness states of individuals, families, or groups in a variety of settings. These skills include history-taking and physical examination skills. Nurses were expected to prepare for these skills in continuing education programs which adhere to ANA approved guidelines, or in baccalaureate nursing programs.

The federal guidelines for nurse practitioner programs define the nurse practitioner as "a registered nurse who has successfully completed a formal program designed to prepare registered nurses to deliver primary health care. . . . "[8]

The geriatric nurse practitioner is defined by the Division on Geriatric Nursing Practice as "a registered nurse who assumes responsibilities of expanding practice in the field of geriatric nursing. . . . The geriatric nurse practitioner is concerned with all stages of health and illness and utilizes knowledge of the aging process in giving and directing care."[9]

The Need for Specialists

Many of the elderly in our population require primary care for chronic disease and health maintenance services. For those who live in long-term care institutions, the problems created by the shortage of physicians is compounded by physicians' reluctance to provide medical care in nursing homes. This reluctance may arise from the fact that the primary care needed by these patients does not fully use the physicians' expertise. Nurse practitioners can fulfill these needs for primary care, furnish the required emotional support, and coordinate related services at a lower cost than physicians can. Further, in many instances, intensive medical care is not always therapeutic, since the goal of care cannot always be cure. Older people with irremedial conditions need assistance in living as fully and comfortably as their disabilities will allow. Primary care is the usual level of care required in nursing homes. Persons requiring secondary care are transferred to hospitals. Persons are admitted to nursing homes because of physical or mental disabilities that interfere severely with the performance of their self-maintenance skills. It is not usually the disease per se that requires their admission to a nursing home but the inability of the person or family members to supplement adequately the person's self-maintenance activities. The person who is not acutely ill but whose death is imminent may remain at home. Therefore, nurses should and must assume much more responsibility for delivering primary care to the elderly in the community as well as in institutions.

Guidelines for Developing Geriatric Nurse Practitioner Programs

Two major sources provide guidelines for the development of nurse practitioner programs or specialist programs in primary care nursing. These are the report to the Secretary of Health, Education and Welfare (HEW), prepared by the Secretary's Committee to Study Extended Roles for Nurses[10] and the description of Nurse Practitioner Training under P.L. 94-63, Title IX, "The Nursing Training Act of 1975."[11] The Secretary's Committee presented their conclusions and recommendations on education, legal considerations, interprofessional relationships between physicians and nurses and their impact on health care delivery; and made definitive and descriptive statements on extended roles for nurses in primary, acute, and long-term care. The description of nurse practitioner training under Title IX includes information on the criteria to be used in evaluating applications for grants to plan, develop, and operate, or significantly expand or maintain existing programs for the training of nurse practitioners. Programs supported by these grants must prepare professional nurses to:

1. assess the health status of individuals and families
2. institute and provide continuity of health care to patients within established protocols
3. provide instruction and counseling to individuals, families, and groups in the areas of health promotion and maintenance
4. work in collaboration with other health care personnel to provide and coordinate services

Other stipulations for these programs require active collaboration between nurses and physicians in the planning, development, and operation of the programs, which must be at least one academic year in length and include both classroom and clinical instruction.

The *Guidelines for Short-Term Continuing Education Programs Preparing the Geriatric Nurse Practitioner*[12] contains a listing of the expected functions of the geriatric nurse practitioner and describes the desirable characteristics of continuing education programs, including goals, organization and administration, faculty, facilities, course content, length of program, and admission and evaluation of students.

In addition to the above guidelines, materials may be obtained on the development of new patterns of collaboration between nurses and physicians—a concept essential to implementing expanded roles for nurses—from the National Joint Practice Commission. This Commission was established by the American Medical Association and the American Nurses' Association to make recommendations for such collaboration of physicians and nurses in order to provide more and better health care to the public. These materials appear to provide sufficient information for the development of nurse practitioner programs.

Problems and Issues

Studies showing the effectiveness of nurse practitioners have been fully reported by Aradine, Bessman, Chappell et al., Charney et al., Duncan et al., Flynn, and Yankauer et al., to list a few,[13-19] and the role of the geriatric nurse practitioner has been amply described in the literature by Heppler, Anderson et al., and Brower et al., among others.[20-22] The litèrature contains descriptions of several continuing education programs for the preparation of geriatric nurse practitioners, including those at the Universities of Colorado, Illinois, and Miami. The need for nurses to assume more responsibility in the delivery of primary care, limitations of nurse practice acts that would prohibit this responsibility, and patient/consumer acceptance of practitioner services do not seem to be considered major issues.

Major issues that have developed seem to revolve around the placement of the educational programs in learning institutions; the difference in length of the various programs; the costs of programs; the speed with which such graduates can be prepared and integrated into existing health services; and finally, appropriate remuneration for these practitioners. The HEW Secretary's Committee to Study Extended Roles for Nurses[23] concluded that, to effect significant changes in the health care system, it would be necessary to prepare over one million active and inactive nurses to function in extended roles, and recommended that sufficient programs in continuing education be set up to produce this large number of nurse practitioners. While continuing education for registered nurses with and without degrees would seem the most likely avenue for this preparation, it is unlikely that sufficient numbers can be prepared quickly enough. The fact that these programs need to be at least one year in length to achieve the objectives presents two difficulties. First, continuing education programs are usually short-term and do not lead to a degree. Many nurses may be expected to desire a degree as a result of this lengthy and rigorous period of study, particularly if they do not already have a degree that is recognized by institutions of higher education. Continuing education programs are expedient for updating nurses and meeting a critical and immediate societal need, but a better long-range approach to the problem of preparing nurses for the expanded role would be to establish programs leading to the master's degree. The baccalaureate degree programs provide both general education and professional preparation at a basic level, a difficult task in itself. Opportunities for professional practice and consolidation of manual and cognitive skills, and application of theory to practice are, of necessity, limited when less than two academic years can be allotted to these functions. Often, this has proven not to be time enough for professional—and in some cases personal—maturation to occur. Consequently, the graduate programs in nursing remain as the most feasible avenue for preparation for expanded roles in nursing. Students in such programs have more professional commitment and experience in making clinical judgments, as well as a level of maturity equivalent to that of professionals in other disciplines.

The second difficulty is the differences in length of programs being offered. This problem is being dealt with through the requirement that, in order to qualify for federal funding, the programs must be discrete and must be at least one academic year in length. Moving the preparation of nurses for extended roles to the graduate level would also serve to decrease the variability in length of programs and would, to some extent, regulate the quality of the programs.

Costs

An *HEW News* release[24] reported on a 15-month study of 44 HEW training and research programs for nurse practitioners and physician assistants. The median cost per graduate ranged from a low of $5,700 for the nurse practitioner with adult care certification, to a high of $15,100 for the physician assistant. This first national analysis of a seven-year effort by HEW revealed that an estimated 5,500 practitioners have been prepared in 145 training and research programs at a cost of more than $50 million. Physician assistant programs ranged from 79 to 104 weeks in length, as compared to 36 to 78 weeks for most nurse practitioner programs. When the physician input in the training programs is high, the cost of such programs is higher than in programs that make greater use of nurse instructors. In our opinion, the question is whether a sufficient number of nurse practitioners can be prepared, even using all the educational resources available. A related question is, How many nurses are interested in accepting responsibility for an expanded role? The answers to these two questions will determine the speed with which we can prepare sufficient numbers of nurse practitioners to affect our health care delivery problems to a significant degree.

Salaries

Appropriate salaries for nurse practitioners may be important as an incentive for nurses to undergo the needed training and to assume added responsibility in the delivery of primary care. Salaries of program graduates have ranged from a low of $13,500 per year for the certified nurse practitioner graduates to a median high of $14,900 per year for nurse practitioners with a Master's degree.[25] Closely related to the matter of salary are the problems arising from attempts to integrate these new practitioners into health services, but the literature reporting on such problems is sparse.

Conclusions

This brief analysis would seem to indicate that while the preparation of nurses for expanded responsibilities in health care is highly desirable, not only for consumers but also for nurses in their search for a stronger professional identity, the effort at present is not powerful enough to have much impact on the health care system. Nevertheless, the movement toward extended roles for nurses in the care of the aged is significant and deserves strong support from educators, administrators, and consumers.

9
Continuing Education in Gerontic Nursing

When social changes and scientific and technological developments are occurring at a rapid pace, continuing education and other lifelong learning opportunities are essential for maintaining high standards of professional practice. The health professionals are particularly vulnerable to obsolescence of knowledge, skill, and even attitudes. To become successful in any occupation, workers need more than knowledge and skills to perform their duties and carry out their responsibilities, more than the minimum educational requirements, more than good health and attractive personality.[1] Workers need to have a commitment to further development of their abilities—both personal and professional. Such commitment usually promotes and sustains enthusiasm, enjoyment, and interest, and may also lead to advancement in work and greater financial rewards. Continuing education is one method of providing opportunities for further personal and professional development.

Nurses as well as other workers are living longer and having longer working careers than previously. Participation in continuing education programs helps nurses to maintain competence and to provide safe and effective care throughout their career lives, thus protecting both clients/patients and themselves as professionals. Much of the psychosocial knowledge being used today in nursing was unknown twenty or thirty years ago. Continuing education can provide a career ladder or the preparation needed to change careers in nursing. For example, it is through continuing education that many nurses are preparing for expanded roles and others are preparing to undertake responsibilities in such specialized areas as neonatal intensive care units and coronary care units.

The American Nurses' Association has established guidelines for state voluntary and mandatory systems of continuing education. Within these guidelines, continuing education is defined as "planned learning experiences beyond a basic nursing education program. These experiences are designed to promote the development of knowledge, skills, and attitudes for the enhancement of nursing practice, thus improving health care to the public."[2]

In-service education is defined as "planned instructional or training programs provided by an employing agency in the work setting and designed to increase competence in a specific area. In-service education is one aspect of continuing education." Staff development is defined as "a total process including both formal and informal learning opportunities. The process is intended to focus on developing the potential of individuals to perform competently in fulfilling their role expectations within a specific agency. Included in the process is orientation, continuing education, and inservice education."

The ANA has established a continuing educational approval and recognition system and developed a set of standards for continuing education. These documents provide ample guides for the development of continuing education programs in nursing.

The ANA code for nurses states, "The nurse maintains individual competence in nursing practice, recognizing and accepting responsibility for individual actions and judgments."[3] It is pointed out that scientific findings, changes in technology and health care services, and expansion of nursing responsibilities can make nursing knowledge obsolete. These changes require nurses to continue to update and expand the body of knowledge on which practice is based through whatever means are appropriate and available, i.e., continuing education, in-service education, staff development, academic study, professional meetings and conferences, reading, workshops, self-assessment reviews, and other methods. Unfortunately, a study in one state has shown that most nurses from all age groups employed and unemployed, were not sufficiently motivated to avoid professional obsolescence through self-directed learning activities.[4]

One of the major functions of institutions of higher education is to provide continuing education and opportunities to the public for lifelong learning. These programs are designed to serve adults of all age groups and to make a variety of educational programs available at times and places convenient for those who desire this instruction. Usually a variety of educational methods are used, such as classroom instruction, televised instruction, correspondence study, seminars, and computer-assisted instruction. The principles of adult learning are used to determine instructional format. In addition, institutions of higher education may provide community service to individuals and groups in order to improve the educational environment of communities, institutions, organizations, and agencies in which adults live, work, and learn.

The academic unit in nursing will usually have some responsibilities for continuing education programs for nurses as well as some responsibility for community service in the form of consultation to nurses working in health agencies.

The Need for Continuing Education

The need for continuing education is a result of constant change.[5] Changes in the health care systems include the present emphasis on primary care, on making health care accessible to all; plans for national health insurance; federal funding for certain segments of the population; reimbursement methods; application of new technologies that create ethical and legal problems as they create the need for new knowledge and skills development and new forms of communication; research promotion that adds responsibilities for nurses to participate in studies, utilize research findings to improve patient care, and conduct research into nursing care problems; new concepts of the team approach and new roles for nurses as team members; and emphasis on quality assurance and cost accountability through peer review processes. Other developments general to all nursing, which increase the need for continuing education, include an emphasis on nursing assessment within the nursing process, the publication of standards for nursing practice, and the implementation of certification procedures and other methods of recognizing outstanding performance in nursing. But most important would seem to be the trend toward mandatory continuing education for relicensure as a method of maintaining professional competency.

The recognition of geriatric nursing as a specialty in nursing by the American Nurses' Association in 1966 provides a specific basis for the need for continuing education in gerontic nursing. Geriatric or gerontic nursing is not required in basic programs that prepare nurses for licensure and has therefore been included in the curriculums of only a few schools of nursing. The American Nurses' Association has been conducting a survey of the extent to which nursing programs have included geriatric nursing since 1975 but the report has not yet been published. Since inclusion of geriatric nursing has not been required by State Boards of Nursing, few nurses have had education in this area. Most nurses, if not all, do, however, have experiences in working with the elderly.

Who Needs Continuing Education?

In planning for the overall nursing care and health needs of people advanced in age, consideration must be given to the preparation of all levels of nursing personnel, beginning with the aide who is not a nurse and who has not had any formal or preservice education and continuing through the level of the registered nurse with doctoral preparation.

The Aide. By far the largest number of personnel providing services for older people in geriatric facilities are aides. The content of a training program suggested for the preparation of aides (see Chapter 4) includes basic personal care skills, selected measures designed to maintain and restore functions, and skills in human relations with special emphasis on the aged and their needs. This instruction may be offered by the university on a demonstration basis in conjunction with programs that prepare nurses to perform in-service education and staff development functions, thus giving in-service education instructor trainees a practical teaching experience.

The Licensed Practical Nurse. Licensed practical nurses constitute the second level of nursing personnel (see Chapter 5). These nurses work under the supervision of the registered nurse or a licensed physician and are prepared to give direct care to patients, including emotional and physical comfort and safety; to record and report patients' conditions; to perform certain specialized nursing functions; and to assist with the rehabilitation of patients according to a plan of care. Continuing education is essential for the practical nurse, regardless of the setting in which she works. It should include instructional material dealing with the social, psychological, and biological aspects of aging in more detail than can be offered in a basic program, with rehabilitative nursing, and—for those who work with terminally ill and dying patients—with some of the psychosocial therapeutic techniques.

The Professional Nurse. The registered nurse is prepared to observe and counsel the ill, injured, or infirm; to maintain health and prevent illness; to identify needs and to develop and implement appropriate plans of nursing care; to supervise and teach other personnel; and to administer therapies, including those prescribed by a licensed physician or dentist. Her performance is based upon knowledge and application of the principles of physical, social, and behavioral sciences. The functions of those who have further prepared themselves as nurse practitioners usually include assessment of the physical and psychosocial health of individuals and families; the use of assessment data to make decisions about treatment in collaboration with physicians and other health professionals; provision of routine health care to patients; evaluation of outcomes of care provided; and the counseling and health teaching of patients and their families. To prepare herself for working with those advanced in age, the nurse practitioner needs additional formal or continuing education in the aging processes and in the techniques and facilities designed for the care of the elderly. Those who work in acute care settings will need some instruction in protecting and caring for the aged in a therapeutic environment.

The Gerontic Nurse Specialist. The highest level of practitioner in nursing is the gerontic nurse specialist, who should be prepared in graduate programs. This specialist will need all the preparation outlined for the nurse practitioner but, in addition, she will need more knowledge of the interaction between health and the aging process; a more extensive foundation for clinical management of patients in stable conditions after diagnosis, treatment, and the prescription of a regimen by the physician or dentist; more advanced intervention strategies; more knowledge and skill in counseling and advising patients and families; more understanding of nursing care problems; more skill in managing an environment for therapeutic purposes; and specialized preparation in managing behavior problems and in the best utilization of nursing resources. Continuing education courses that are designed to keep all these knowledges and skills updated are as essential for the gerontic nurse specialist, as are the courses designed for nursing personnel at staff level. The gerontic nurse specialist may further specialize and prepare to function as a long-term care specialist who cares for sick and disabled individuals who are maintained in residential facilities and who need nursing care, instruction in self-care, and—along with their families—instruction in rehabilitative techniques. Others may want to prepare to function as gerontic health nurse specialists to work with normal, healthy aged members of the community who need health teaching about prevention and the maintenance of a high level of physical and mental functioning; or ambulatory patients who need continuing surveillance of existing health problems, access to a variety of medical and health services, and all levels of preventive care.

The Nurse Gerontologist. There is also the need for some nurses to have preparation in gerontology at the doctoral level so that they may apply the knowledge of gerontology to the study of the interaction between health and the aging processes, and to the solution of care problems for those advanced in age. Nursing knowledge at present does not adequately provide for the continued advancement of nursing practice in the care of the aged. Further, applied research is needed to assist the gerontic nurse specialist to deal adequately with personal and psychological care, the management of social and interpersonal relationships, the provision of therapeutic environments, and the preparation of nursing personnel for their particular jobs. Researchers need to keep their knowledges and skills updated as methods and techniques change and new concepts develop.

Content of Continuing Education Courses

Three important sources from which topics and content for continuing education courses in gerontic nursing may be derived are publications of the ANA: *Standards for Gerontological Nursing Practice;*[6] *Guidelines for Short-Term Continuing Education Programs Preparing the Geriatric Nurse Practitioner;*[7] and *Geriatric Nursing Certification.*[8]

In 1976 the National League for Nursing developed a short-term instruction program and an instructors' guide for a course for licensed practical nurses employed in nursing homes.[9,10] These materials were designed to increase the nurse's knowledge of the social aspects of care rather than knowledge of the procedures related to the illness. There are sections in both guides on observation, assessment, care planning, and evaluation.

Also available are topical outlines for baccalaureate and graduate courses in the nursing care of the elderly, materials on legislative developments; published guidelines from various sources; and suggestions from nursing personnel.

At a workshop on continuing education for gerontic nurses conducted at The Pennsylvania State University in August, 1975, participants, all of whom were registered nurses employed in agencies whose clients were age 55 or over, were asked to complete a questionnaire about what competencies (knowledge, skills, attitudes) are most critically needed by the aide, the licensed practical nurse, the nursing student, and the registered nurse in gerontic nursing. Thirty-nine questionnaires were completed. The following list, compiled from data obtained by the questionnaire, identifies these needs and also demonstrates the overlap of needs among the various categories of personnel:

1. Aging process
    a. emotional, psychological, and physiological changes
    b. behavioral limitations
2. Legal aspects
    a. state and federal regulations governing facilities
    b. documentation in nursing records
3. Professional ethics and skills
    a. role delineation
    b. respect for line of authority
    c. tact in dealing with family
4. Environmental effects
    a. geographical and cultural changes
5. Fundamental nursing skills
    a. bathing and hygiene
    b. prevention
        1. skin breakdown
        2. contractures
        3. fluid and electrolyte balance
    c. body mechanics (lifting and transfer)
    d. importance of individualized care
        1. accepting patient as individual
        2. allowing independence
6. Communication—both verbal and nonverbal (listening)
    a. patient, family and staff
7. Rehabilitation
    a. restorative skills—range of motion
    b. reality orientation
8. Patience; empathy
9. Dealing with death and dying
    a. Basic patterns of need which were found specific to each level of nursing were:
        1. Nurse Aide

        a. staying within limits of role
        b. technical skills
        c. accepting patient as individual
        d. accepting patients' limitations
    2. Licensed Practical Nurse (same for nursing student and registered nurse)
        a. nursing care of whole patient
            1. medication administration and pharmacology of drugs used
            2. procedures (treatments, use of equipment)
            3. knowledge of community resources
            4. observation of patient to perceive needs
        b. management skills
            1. oversee ancillary staff
                a. aide
                b. orderly
    3. Nursing Student
        a. orientation to facility
            1. health care
            2. meet staff
            3. policies and procedures, philosophy of faculty
        b. use of nursing process
            1. assess patient and identify needs
            2. develop and implement plan
        c. awareness of self—understanding self and others
        d. health teaching for patients
            1. disease processes
            2. medications—use and adverse effects
            3. accept own limitations
        e. attitude—assist the student to realize need for R.N. in geriatrics
    4. Registered Nurse
        a. change agent—engender positive attitude toward change
        b. to be an effective geriatric nurse
            1. keep abreast of new developments in geriatrics

    2. update knowledge of staff
       a. nursing skills
       b. medications
       c. terminology
       d. resources available—medicare, medicaide
    3. apply research to improve quality of care
  c. administrative duties
    1. motivate staff and utilize all available nursing skills
    2. promote professional ethics among staff
    3. promote adherence to regulations of facility
    4. assess patient care—quality, efficiency

The foregoing list, or any of the sources discussed here, can be used in planning topics and content for continuing education courses and in formulating an overall design to cover the field, which is necessary to assure that a comprehensive body of knowledge can be presented within a specified period of time. Such a plan will also help to avoid the tendency to plan content based on current interests or fads. The need is to instruct nurses in geriatric facilities who have not had previous formal preparation in this area, as well as to teach these nurses the latest knowledge, skills, and attitudes.

Program Format for Continuing Education Programs

The principles guiding the construction of the format for continuing education programs are based on knowledge of adult development and learning. Some of this knowledge is best obtained through university courses offered by schools or colleges of education. One very useful book is *The Process of Staff Development* by Tobin et al.,[11] which contains discussions of the concepts, philosophy, purpose, and goals for continuing education, in-service education, and staff development; history of staff development in nursing; guidelines for adult learning; how to identify learner needs, how to design and implement programs, select teaching methods, and evaluate outcomes. Two other important sources relating to continuing education in nursing in general are the ANA Council on Continuing Education and the *Journal of Continuing Education in Nursing*.

An article on facilitating staff learning, based on a training module developed in a gerontology manpower training project,[12] suggests techniques for overcoming adult learning problems such as anxiety, memory problems, physical difficulties, loss of speed in performance, goal orientation, and lack of motivation. An abstract of the article follows.

Teaching Mature Adults

1. Respect the adult student's prior experience—his primary goal is *not* the role of student
2. To alleviate the anxiety which most adults experience when entering the classroom situation:
    a. begin by getting acquainted; introduce yourself and give the group an opportunity to get to know you and each other
    b. encourage questions and other verbal contributions by reinforcing comments and questions in a *positive* manner
3. Expect a broad range of individual differences in intellectual ability
    a. be prepared to repeat instructions
    b. encourage questions
    c. avoid use of jargon
4. To jog memories:
    a. cue redundantly; repeat the same message in a number of ways, e.g., say it and write it on the chalkboard at the same time
    b. encourage note taking
    c. define obscure words and phrases
    d. encourage the group to verbalize concepts and draw conclusions, and to relate personal experience to classroom concepts
    e. A written outline of the presentation will be helpful to the student in relating parts of the whole to each other

5. To help compensate for physical impairments such as sensory loss (which are more likely to occur in an adult group):
   a. speak slightly louder than you would in ordinary conversation
   b. enunciate clearly; do not speak in a monotone
   c. face the group as much as possible when speaking
   d. repeat questions and comments from the group so that all may hear
   e. use large letters when writing on the chalkboard
   f. make certain the classroom is well lighted
   g. allow time for rest breaks

Not all these techniques will apply in all situations, but they are presented here in the hope that they might be useful should the need arise.

To make group discussions more fruitful, material from another article from the Gerontology Center may be most useful.[13]

In the specific area of gerontic nursing, a guide to in-service education for nursing personnel in nursing homes has been prepared by Mayne.[14] It provides a simple yet basic outline for program development but does not describe specific content in the area of long-term care. Ernest's[15] in-service educator's guide for training residents/clients, family members, board members, volunteers, and nursing staff considers the characteristics of the aged population and age changes in vision, hearing, touch, dexterity, taste, smell, and mobility and balance. This manual also describes the principles of in-service training and includes a few pertinent but simple principles of adult education such as:

> People are more likely to learn by doing.
> Learning is easier if the student is ready to learn.
> Using what the student already knows can speed learning.
> It is easier to learn one thing at a time rather than many complicated procedures.
> Understanding what is to be learned is a basic process in education.
> Practice of the procedures until understanding has taken place is essential.
> People learn at different rates.

Four other training modules were developed by participants in the project conducted at The Pennsylvania State University. Volume I, prepared by Hickey and Fatula,[16] contains descriptions of programmed training modules on gerontology, including general training instructions, a discussion of sensory deprivation and the elderly, appendixes, and reference notes. These authors hold that the primary objective of sensory deprivation training is the improvement of social interactions between the care-giver trainee and the elderly. Content includes such topics as changes in sensory modalities, environmental adaptation, territoriality, and proxemics. The three units of the module require about three hours for completion and can be used for heterogeneous groups as large as thirty. Course material may be presented by the videotape "Make a Wish,"* which was prepared for use with this module to enhance trainees' awareness of sensory loss; by lecture; by demonstration by a seasoned practitioner; or through the use of devices which simulate loss of hearing or sight and give insight into problems resulting from sensory impairment.

Zerbe and Hickey[17] prepared Volume II, which presents a module of six programmed units for a continuing education program in gerontology. This module deals primarily with self-maintenance skills for the elderly. It not only supplies the health worker with theoretical and practical knowledge about the aging process and the aging patient, but also provides the teaching vehicle (behavior modification) through which this knowledge can be applied to real-life situations in the work area. All health care personnel who deal with the physical care of elderly persons can benefit by participating in a program that utilizes this module. The module contains a content outline for the instructor, who should be either a registered nurse or a health-related person already trained in the principles of basic care for the elderly and have some background in behavior modification theory.

Volume III, by Greenberg et al.,[18] is composed of programmed training modules on gerontology that deal primarily with verbal and nonverbal communication skills for the gerontologic practitioner. The program contained in the module consists

*Available from The Pennsylvania State University, College of Human Development, University Park, Pa. 16802.

of five two-hour sessions all of which must be attended since they are sequenced. Because of its versatility, this training module can be used with trainees of varying educational levels. However, the program is most applicable to participants with some college and/or vocational training (L.P.N.s and R.N.s). Groups should not exceed fifteen participants. The instructor should be someone with experience in communication problems and it is important that the trainer have some educational background and knowledge in the field of aging.

Volume IV, prepared by Hickey and his coworkers,[19] is a series of programmed training modules on gerontology that contain material on loss reaction and grief management. This module was designed to train service workers to deal more effectively with the dying, especially terminally ill patients, and the bereaved. It consists of six two-hour sessions on varying topics related to dying, death, and bereavement. Between 15 and 32 trainees can be accommodated by this module. Each session consists of a presentation by tape, film, or filmstrip, and/or lecture, followed by discussion in small groups of five participants. The instructor should be an experienced teacher.

Current Issues Relating to Continuing Education

Should continuing education for nurses be mandatory? This is one of the serious issues in nursing today. Many adverse criticisms of professional licensure stem from the fact that professionals usually undergo only one examination to practice and may renew a license for a lifetime by merely paying a fee at intervals, thus making it possible for incompetent practitioners to continue to practice. The Federal government has become increasingly involved in supporting health services for certain segments of the population but has no way of guaranteeing that the services provided are of high quality. As a result, pressure from governmental sources that there be evidence of continuing education as a requirement for relicensure is increasing. Some nurses are resisting this trend because continuing education courses are not easily available to all segments of the nursing population. They also ask, "Who should finance continuing education?" Some think it unfair to pass these costs along to the consumers of health services, yet many nurses insist that they cannot afford to take time off from work without pay, in addition to paying the costs for the course, travel, and other expenses. Some nurses say they keep their skills and knowledge updated through practice, but, on the other hand, there is evidence that some of these nurses do not belong to professional associations, subscribe to journals, attend conferences, or take responsibility for continued learning, which is necessary to maintain a satisfactory level of performance.

Objections to mandatory requirement of continuing education have been summarized.[20] These include the difficulty of assessing learning, particularly in continuing education; the fact that people can attend courses without learning; the lack of evidence that these courses bring about better performance; the cost; limitation of resources; the system of record keeping; and the difficulty of accrediting and evaluating the program offered. Others believe that the individual's commitment and responsibility play a part in determining the effectiveness of continuing education.[21] They also point out the difficulties confronting nurses who try to change clinical situations when they have learned new ways of approaching clinical problems and implementing new knowledge.

Evaluation of continuing education in terms of its contribution to the improvement of nursing practice is an important current issue. At the present time there are no documented studies to show that nurses who take continuing education courses provide a higher quality of care than those who do not take such courses. Even though an examination of certification credentials would indicate that nurses who have had courses in gerontology and the nursing care of the elderly provide the best documentation, evidence of improvement in performance has yet to be subjected to scientific study. Perhaps the question of effectiveness should be answered before continuing education is made mandatory for relicensure.

Another issue is related to the different kinds of continuing education needed for nurses fulfilling different roles in nursing, i.e., teachers, administrators, researchers, and specialists, as well as practicing nurses at the staff level. Most programs offered at the present time are one-day conferences or workshops offered to nurses at all levels, and are not planned in such a way that one builds on another. Too often programs consist of material that relates to popular current topics, e.g., sexuality, death, and dying. What is needed is a comprehensive approach to continuing education programs in each area so that nurses may develop a growing expertise or even develop a specialization in an area. Also, employers need to be willing to allow at least two people to attend a particular program so they can support each other in consulting with their coworkers on their return to the job and in implementing new concepts and changes.

Evaluation of the effectiveness of continuing education is particularly difficult for the sponsoring agency since it may require follow-up of students from a wide geographical area and contact with numerous widely scattered agencies in which the nurses practice. It would also entail some responsibility on the part of the employing agencies since nurses' performance would have to be evaluated in relation to the continuing education offerings. Further, it is realized that a nurse's performance is the function of many variables. However, given the many issues involved, it is still realized that continuing education and staff development are essential if quality care is to be provided and professional obsolescence is to be prevented.

Recommendations

From the foregoing discussion and from the author's experiences in the area of continuing education for gerontic nurses, the following recommendations are made:

1. Institutions that sponsor continuing education programs in gerontic nursing should develop a long-range and comprehensive plan for delivering the content needed for improving prac-

tice in this specialized area. This is particularly important since the curriculums for generic programs have no requirements in geriatric nursing. Instead of offering a large number of different programs in one year, a smaller number could be offered and repeated in different localities. These courses, with appropriate updating, might be repeated again in five years or at suitable intervals. An entirely new schedule of courses would be offered the second year, and repeated in five years, and so on.

These long-range plans of course offerings should be made available to nurses and health agencies so that nurses could know about them and assume responsibility for their own professional development.

2. The continuing education needs of nurses practicing at advanced levels differ from those of nurses at other levels, and careful consideration should be given to these needs. Since there are fewer of these nurses, and a dearth of qualified faculty in specialized areas, perhaps state, regional, or national professional associations would be in the best position to provide this costly type of education at lower cost than local agencies could provide it, under some mechanism that would be similar in concept to an academy.

Consideration also needs to be given to the amount and kind of continued education needed by nurses in different roles. For example, it might be more beneficial for nurse researchers to attend scientific meetings than to take a course through continuing education.

3. Nurses should be encouraged to utilize continuing education offerings in other disciplines which underlie or relate to nursing practice; for example, gerontology, psychology, sociology, education, business administration, to name a few.

4. Nurses should be encouraged to maintain curriculum vitae or portfolios of their educational and professional experiences and achievements, not only for their own use in planning for systematic career development, but for use by employing agencies in their selection of personnel. Many employers of nurses place each nurse employed at the beginning salary level without regard to her preparation, experience, or achievement, a fact which lessens greatly the incentive for nurses to pursue the

development of their careers to the fullest extent possible. So far, there has been no reward for the time, effort, and money required for the systematic development of a career except earned formal educational credentials.

5. Research must be done to clarify the relations of continuing education, in-service education, and staff development to performance and, most important, to measures for determining effectiveness in terms of improvement in patient care. Also, there needs to be greater emphasis on the utilization in practice of the research findings now available.

6. Nurses need to be encouraged to see the potential of using knowledge and skills in multiple settings, since most gerontic nursing knowledge is applicable, perhaps with some adaptations or modifications, in any setting.

7. A compendium of the various available training modules and manuals should be compiled so as to be more readily accessible to teachers and other consumers. (Many of these manuals are currently available in mimeograph form only.)

8. Finally, careful consideration needs to be given to reexamination for relicensure as possibly a more feasible method than mandatory continuing education to assure the competence of professional practitioners. Then nurses could prepare for relicensure by whatever means would be most feasible for their life and learning styles, and examinations could be prepared that might reflect preparation for special areas of practice more precisely than would enrollment for a specific number of continuing education credits.

Appendix A
A Guide to Content Analysis for Computer-Based Nursing Courses

Content Category	Symbol	Definition	Examples
Fact	F	Specific information describing "what actually is" or "what actually has been"	Banting and Best discovered insulin. One gram equals 15 grains. Washington is the capital of the United States.
Supposition	S	Statements in which what is *claimed* to be is presented as if it were fact	The personality is made up of the id, the ego, and the superego. (Note that if the statement read, "In psychoanalytic theory, the personality is represented as consisting of the id, the ego, and the superego," this would constitute a *fact* in this system of content analysis.)

(continued)

Appendix A (continued)

Content Category	Symbol	Definition	Examples
Concept	(see below)	*Category* or *class* of different objects, persons, events, etc., that share at least some common characteristics despite their differences	
Concept Name	CN	Label used to designate a concept	*Accident* is a label applied to a category of events. *Registered nurse* is a label applied to a category of persons. *Parasympathetic* is a label applied to a category of nerves.
Concept Definition	CD	A statement of the denotative meaning of a concept label (i.e., the dictionary definition)	*Parasympathetic* nerves comprise the system of peripheral autonomic nerves that have their origin in the brain stem and sacral spinal cord.
Concept Features	CF	The distinctive attributes or characteristics of a concept.	*Parasympathetic* nervous system: 1. craniosacral origin 2. ganglia near effector organs 3. preganglionic fibers long 4. postganglionic fibers short 5. neuroeffector transmitter acetylcholine, etc.
Concept Example	CE	An instance or exemplar that has the distinctive features of the concept	*Vagus nerve* is an example of the concept *parasympathetic*.

Concept Nonexample	NCE	An instance or exemplar that does not have the distinctive features of the concept	The *sciatic nerve* is a nonexample of the concept *parasympathetic*.
Principle	(see below)	A verifiable generalization about the relationship of two or more concepts	
Principle Definition	PD	A statement describing the relationship of two or more concepts (can often be expressed by "If . . . then" statements)	*Parasympathetic* stimulation results in energy conservation reactions. (*If* parasympathetic stimulation, *then* energy conservation.)
Principle Example	PE	A specific instance of the operation of a principle	Stimulation of the vagus nerve results in slowing of the heart rate.
Dictum	D	A rule for action based on opinion or judgment; lacks the verification of a principle	First aid in suicide prevention is directed to counteracting hopelessness.

Appendix B
A Course Model for
Computer-based Instruction

These computer-based courses have been prepared by authors from the faculty of the Nursing Department at The Pennsylvania State University, guided by a course model composed of an instruction sequence and a comprehensive final examination. The instruction sequence in a computer-based course can incorporate a variety of methods, materials, and activities, and can be classified on a continuum of computer utilization ranging from Computer Managed Instruction (CMI) to Computer Assisted Instruction (CAI). At the CAI extreme is the tutorial course where all instruction is done "on-line," that is, at a computer terminal. At the CMI end of the continuum, all instruction consists of self-study modules of instruction that are presented "off-line," using printed material, slides, audio tapes, etc., that are not under computer control. These "off-line" materials, selected by authors on the basis of course objectives, are grouped into the basic unit of instruction—a lesson. Coherent lessons are subsumed under a larger unit of instruction called a module. In CMI, the use of the computer for instruction (over and above pre- and posttesting) is restricted to presentation at the end of each lesson of questions designed to serve three purposes: 1. to assess comprehension of the lesson material; 2. to provide a basis for prescribing remedial study; and 3. to stimulate the learner to engage in the active cognitive processing prerequisite for learning. Such a computer-based study management system, based on modern cognitive learning theory, has been reported by Anderson et al.[1] at the University of Illinois.

The comprehensive final examination consists of test items randomly sampled from a pool generated from each lesson of the course. Performance records are grouped into subtests for each module of instruction. In order to complete the course satisfactorily, the student must reach criterion (the cutoff score for a test or subtest) not only on the total examination, but on each of the modular subtests. Remedial instruction and reexamination are provided on modules when performance is below standards set by the faculty. Even though the student is tested within each lesson, a comprehensive final examination is included because it is believed that it measures some aspects of learning, and clues to appropriate remedial instruction are obtainable only by a comprehensive test.

Computer Managed Review and Examination in Nursing 310: Nursing Care of the Elderly*

Course Outline

A. Description:
  1. Nursing 310: Nursing Care of the Elderly
  2. Prerequisites: Nursing 215, 225, 230, IFS 349
  3. Credits: 5
  4. Course Description:
     Nursing 310 has as its focus the person in the latter stages of the developmental continuum of life, and as its aim, the expansion of the student's capabilities in utilizing the nursing process, and in communicating and cooperating

*Prepared by Carmen A. Estes and Carolyn Cuffey at The Pennsylvania State University Department of Nursing, College of Human Development Computer Assisted Instruction Laboratory, College of Education. October, 1975.

with other health care workers, to provide nursing care for elderly individuals with selected health problems.
B. Objectives:
At the completion of the course, it is expected that the student will be able to:
1. Describe the basic tenets of at least two developmental views of aging, and a variety of developmental tasks of the aged and their nursing implications
2. Compare normal physiological and psychosocial functioning in the aged with those at other developmental levels
3. Compare pathophysiological and psychosocial manifestations of disease in the aged with those at other developmental levels
4. Identify relationships between processes associated with aging, the problems and needs of the elderly, and their response to stress and to health care
5. Identify and describe selected health problems frequently found among the elderly in our society
6. Utilize previous learning in formulating nursing care for the elderly person aimed at promoting, maintaining, and restoring health
7. Demonstrate ability to provide nursing care for the elderly patient with selected health problems by
   a. identifying and classifying relevant assessment data
   b. identifying appropriate nursing care objectives and evaluative criteria
   c. selecting appropriate nursing interventions
   d. comparing outcomes of interventions with the evaluative criteria in order to make judgments regarding their effectiveness
   e. modifying the plan of care in the light of changing patient problems and needs, the accretion of assessment data, and the effectiveness of interventions
C. Textbooks:
1. Bergersen, B., and Sakalys, J. *Review of Pharmacology in Nursing*. St. Louis: C. V. Mosby Co., 1974.
2. Browning, M. H. (comp). *Nursing and the Aging Patient*.

Contemporary Nursing Series. New York: The American Journal of Nursing Co., 1974.
3. Estes, C., and Cuffey, C. (comp.). *Computer Managed Review and Examination: Nursing Care of the Elderly.* University Park, Pa.: The Pennsylvania State University, October, 1975.
4. Moidel, H. C., Sorensen, G. E., Gilbin, E. C., and Kaufman, M. A. (eds.). *Nursing Care of the Patient with Medical-Surgical Disorders.* New York: McGraw-Hill Book Co., 1971.

D. Library References:
1. Burnside, I. M. (ed.). *Psychosocial Nursing Care of the Aged.* New York: McGraw-Hill Book Co., 1973.
2. Cowdry, E. V., and Steinberg, F. U. (eds.). *The Care of the Geriatric Patient.* (4th ed.) St. Louis: C. V. Mosby Co., 1971.
3. Erikson, E. *Childhood and Society.* (2nd ed.) New York: W. W. Norton & Co., 1963.
4. Havighurst, R. J. *Developmental Tasks and Education.* (3rd ed.) New York: David McKay Co., 1972.

Topic Outline

Nursing 310: Nursing Care of the Elderly

Module A: PERSPECTIVES ON AGING
    Lesson 1   Erikson: developmental stages; nursing applications of Erikson
    Lesson 2   Havighurst: developmental tasks
    Lesson 3   Implications of geriatric nursing practice standard relevant to dying and death

Module B: DIMENSIONS OF AGING
    Lesson 1   Overview of selected aspects of aging: physiological changes, sensory changes, environmental impact, effects of institutionalization, social behavior changes, etc.

	Lesson 2	Psychological aspects of aging: independence, fears, effects of losses in support systems
	Lesson 3	Nursing implications of decreasing behavioral pace in the elderly
	Lesson 4	Loneliness of old age
	Lesson 5	Nursing assessment based on knowledge of developmental level; nursing intervention to maintain functional capacity; relevance of geriatric nursing practice standard
	Lesson 6	Communication and social interaction in aged
Module C:	GERIATRIC NURSING	
	Lesson 1	Brief history of geriatric nursing
	Lesson 2	Standards for geriatric nursing practice
	Lesson 3	Role of professional nurse in health maintenance
	Lesson 4	Role of professional nurse in rehabilitation
	Lesson 5	Major aspects of Medicare
Module D:	PSYCHOLOGICAL DYSFUNCTION; BEHAVIOR PROBLEMS	
	Lesson 1	Assessment and nursing interventions in problems related to confusion
	Lesson 2	Psychiatric aspects of geriatrics
	Lesson 3	Nursing goals and interventions: aged psychiatric patient
	Lesson 4	Suicide as a problem
	Lesson 5	Psychotropic drugs: major and minor tranquilizers
Module E:	METABOLIC PROBLEMS	
	Lesson 1	Diabetes mellitus: pathophysiology, management
	Lesson 2	Coping with hypoglycemic reactions
	Lesson 3	Diabetes mellitus in the aged
	Lesson 4	Drugs: insulin, oral hypoglycemic agents

Module F: GASTROINTESTINAL PROBLEMS
- Lesson 1 Aging GI system; manifestations and management of GI problems common in the elderly
- Lesson 2 Nutritional problems of the elderly
- Lesson 3 Stomach disorders: nursing care
- Lesson 4 Intestinal disorders: nursing care
- Lesson 5 Long-term care of the patient with cancer
- Lesson 6 Drugs: antacids, antidiarrheics, cathartics

Module G: NEUROLOGICAL PROBLEMS
- Lesson 1 Sensory losses; devices to maintain and enhance functional abilities; implications of relevant geriatric nursing standard
- Lesson 2 Cerebrovascular disorders in later life
- Lesson 3 Nursing care of the stroke patient
- Lesson 4 Nursing care of the brain-damaged patient
- Lesson 5 Parkinson's syndrome
- Lesson 6 Antiparkinsonism drugs

Module H: UROLOGICAL PROBLEMS
- Lesson 1 Aging genitourinary system; common renal problems in the elderly
- Lesson 2 Kidney disorders: nursing care
- Lesson 3 Common lower urinary tract problems in the elderly
- Lesson 4 Lower tract problems: nursing care
- Lesson 5 Nursing problems with indwelling catheter

Module I: CARDIOVASCULAR PROBLEMS
- Lesson 1 Ischemic heart disease: nursing care
- Lesson 2 Heart failure: nursing care
- Lesson 3 Congestive heart failure: early recognition, pulmonary edema, diuretic therapy
- Lesson 4 Arrhythmias: general nursing care

	Lesson 5	Aging cardiovascular system; heart diseases in the elderly
	Lesson 6	Cardiovascular drugs: glycosides, quinidine, anticoagulants, nitroglycerin
Module J:	PERIPHERAL VASCULAR PROBLEMS	
	Lesson 1	Peripheral vascular disease in the elderly: general nursing implications.
	Lesson 2	Peripheral vascular disease: surgical intervention, prostheses, nursing implications
	Lesson 3	Pulmonary embolism
Module K:	BRONCHOPULMONARY PROBLEMS	
	Lesson 1	Aging respiratory system
	Lesson 2	Respiration in emphysema
	Lesson 3	Impact of emphysema
Module L:	MUSCULOSKELETAL PROBLEMS	
	Lesson 1	Muscular changes with aging; common disorders in aged
	Lesson 2	Skeletal problems in aging: osteoporosis
	Lesson 3	Skeletal injuries in aged
	Lesson 4	Nursing in internal hip fixation
	Lesson 5	Joint diseases in the elderly: arthritis
	Lesson 6	Total hip replacement: nursing care
	Lesson 7	Drugs: analgesic-antipryetic-analgesics, phenylbutazone, indomethacin

Introduction and General Directions

The *CMRE Handbook* contains information that is essential for Computer Managed Review and Examination.

The first thing the handbook provides is an overview of this course. It provides you with the general scope and objectives of the course, the major topics that are considered, and a specific topic outline.

Following the topic outline, you will see listed the sources in which study materials are located. These sources include required texts, (available for purchase by the student), library reference books (available under specified loan conditions), and, finally, this handbook itself. The body of the *CMRE Handbook* is your guide to the specific reading material for every study prescription in this course. There is a page in this handbook for every reference located in either a student text or a library reference book. On each page appears the name of the author of the reference, the title, the source, the page numbers, and the location where it may be found. For some references, the actual reading material is contained in this handbook.

Handbook pages are numbered with a code called a "prescription code." If you look at the course outline you will see that CMRE courses are divided into a number of modules and each module is divided into several lessons. Each lesson has one or more articles, excerpts from textbooks, etc. Each reference has one or more pages of reading material. Look at the following example from Nursing 310.

Module A: PERSPECTIVES ON AGING
          Lesson 1   Erikson, E. Youth and the life cycle . . . p. 43.
                        Erikson, E. Ego integrity vs. despair . . . pp. 268–269
                        Bancroft, A. Integrity and despair . . . pp. 129–136
          Lesson 2   Havighurst, R. J. Developmental tasks . . . pp. 107–116
          Lesson 3   Davis, B. Until death ensues . . . pp. 303–309
                        Kavanaugh, R. Helping patients . . . facing death . . . pp. 35–42

If you look at the example you can see that Module A has three lessons. Lesson 1 has three references, Lesson 2 has 1 reference, and Lesson 3 has 2 references. The handbook page numbers for the article by Bancroft would thus be:

A: 1: 3
Module / Lesson / Reference

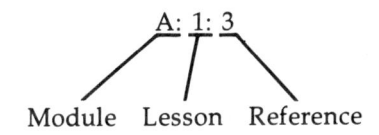

The full prescription code for the Bancroft article is:

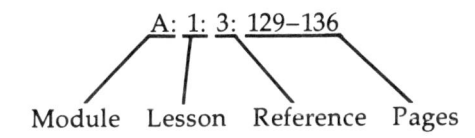

A: 1: 3: 129–136
Module / Lesson / Reference / Pages

A full explanation of prescription codes is available to you on the computer when you begin the CMRE course.

In summary, if you want to know what a course is about, what to study, and where to find it, you can find the answer in your handbook.

Table of Contents

INTRODUCTIONS AND GENERAL DIRECTIONS vii

COURSE OUTLINE FOR NURSING 310 ix
A. Description ix
B. Objectives ix
C. Textbooks ix
D. Library References ix

TOPIC OUTLINE FOR NURSING 310 xi

REQUIRED READINGS:
The Eight Stages in the Life Cycle of Man A:1:1
Childhood and Society A:1:2
Integrity and Despair: A Contrast of Two Lives A:1:3
Developmental Tasks and Education A:2:1
Until Death Ensues A:3:1
Helping Patients Who Are Facing Death A:3:2
Caring for the Aged B:1:1
Psychologic Aspects of Geriatric Nursing B:2:1
Give the Older Person Time B:3:1

The Loneliness of Old Age B:4:1
Assessing Behavior in the Elderly B:5:1
Communication and Social Interaction in the Aged B:6:1
Coming of Age: A Challenge for Geriatric Nursing C:1:1
Standards for Geriatric Nursing Practice C:2:1
The Role of a Professional Nurse in a
  Health Maintenance Program C:3:1
The Rehabilitation Process C:4:1
Later Developments: Medicine,
  Social Sciences, and Nursing C:4:2
What is Medicare C:5:1
Guidelines for the Care of Confused Patients D:1:1
Care of the Confused Elderly Patient D:1:2
Psychiatric Aspects D:2:1
The Aged Psychiatric Patient D:3:1
When Words Fail D:3:2
Preventing Suicide D:4:1
Suicide in the Aged D:4:2
Major Tranquilizers: Minor Tranquilizers D:5:1
Diabetes Mellitus E:1:1
Coping with the Complex, Dangerous, Elusive Problem of
  Those Insulin-induced Hypoglycemic Reactions E:2:1
Diabetes Mellitus in the Aged E:3:1
Hormones of the Pancreas and Oral Hypoglycemic Agents . E:4:1
Gastrointestinal Diseases in the Aged F:1:1
It's Not Age that Interferes with Nutrition
  of the Elderly F:2:1
Disorders of the Stomach F:3:1
Adenocarcinoma F:4:1
Better Techniques for Bagging Stomas F:4:2
Long-term Care of the Patient with Cancer F:5:1
Drugs Affecting the Gastrointestinal System F:6:1
Accoutrements of Aging G:1:1
Cerebrovascular Disorders in Later Life G:2:1
Nursing Care of the Stroke Patient G:3:1
Adapting Care for the Brain-damaged Patient G:4:1
Basal Ganglia, Parkinson's Syndrome G:5:1
Antiparkinsonism Drugs G:5:2

Medical Renal Diseases in the Aged H:1:1
Infections of the Urinary Tract H:2:1
Common Lower Urinary Tract Problems in Older Persons . H:3:1
Cystitis, Obstruction, Urinary Calculi H:4:1
Nursing Problem: Bacteriuria and the
    Indwelling Catheter H:5:1
Coronary Artery Disease I:1:1
Clinical Syndromes of Heart Failure I:2:1
Early Signs of Congestive Heart Failure I:3:1
Acute Pulmonary Edema I:3:2
Complications of Diuretic Therapy I:3:3
Nursing Care of Patients with Arrhythmias I:4:1
Special Features of Heart Disease in the
    Elderly Patients I:5:1
Cardiovascular Drugs I:6:1
The Elderly Person with Peripheral Vascular Problems ... J:1:1
Foot Welfare J:1:2
The Elderly Person with Peripheral Vascular Problems ... J:2:1
Pulmonary Embolism J:3:1
Respiratory System K:1:1
Prevalent Pulmonary Diseases in the Aged K:1:2
Respiration in Emphysema Patients K:2:1
The Impact of Emphysema K:3:1
Why Emphysema Patients Are the Way They Are K:3:2
Common Disorders of Muscles in the Aged L:1:1
Metabolic Disorders of the Skeleton in Aging L:2:1
Injuries to the Skeletal System of Older Persons L:3:1
Nursing the Patient with Internal Hip Fixation L:4:1
Prevalent Joint Diseases in Older Persons L:5:1
Total Hip Replacement L:6:1
Drugs that Affect the Central Nervous System L:7:1

Appendix C
A Course Outline for Gerontic Nursing

Course:
490.3 Gerontic Nursing
Credit Hours:
5-10
Class Hours/week 1
Laboratory Hours 20-36
Prerequisites:
11th Term Standing (Students have had a required introductory course in gerontic nursing)

Course Objectives:
1. The student should develop an awareness of his own and societal attitudes toward aging.
2. The student should develop skill in various assessment methods and techniques.
3. The student should be able to describe and/or define the kind and degree of physiological and sociological changes associated with aging based on the literature, discussions, and observations of aging persons.
4. The student should understand the scientific and humanistic concepts of the normal aging process.
5. The student should use the ANA geriatric nursing standards to plan, implement, and evaluate nursing care for the aged.

Overview of Content:
I. Use of attitude scales in the understanding of individual and societal attitudes toward aging.
II. Assessment methods and techniques
III. Changes associated with aging
IV. ANA geriatric standards

Teaching Methods:
Students will have patients assigned to them for all aspects of nursing care and will be encouraged to participate in all discussions related to the patients and their families. Special rounds and conferences will be held with students. In addition, students will be encouraged to take part in clinical staff conferences and other aspects of the regular in-service education programs.

Learning activities may include:
1. Independent study under computer managed instruction
2. Case studies
3. Nursing assessments
4. Nursing care plan audits
5. Conferences with the instructor
6. Abstracts of articles on geriatric nursing used in providing care
7. Book review of a textbook on nursing the aged
8. Use of a variety of nursing forms such as nursing history, activities of daily living, coordinated health services form, etc.
9. Written descriptions of experiences in practice settings
10. Written discussion of the value of the various forms used
11. Written discussion on the use of ANA Standards for Geriatric Nursing Practice

Evaluations:
The students' evaluation will consist of a self-evaluation, instructor's evaluation of course assignments, and an evaluation by the nurse/nurses in the facility where the student is assigned for practice.

Appendix D
A Sample of a Short-term Training Program

The following materials are used to illustrate a short-term continuing education program funded by the Public Health Traineeship Program administered by a Regional Office of the Public Health Service. The objectives of these short-term traineeship grants were

> (a) to assist in increasing the substantive technical competence of professional health personnel by enabling them to update their knowledge and skills relating to the public health programs in which they are engaged, and (b) to decrease the time lag between the discovery of new knowledge in the field of public health and its effective application in public health practice."[1]

Project Abstract

Project Title:
Update (II) Knowledge and Skills of Registered Nurses Who Serve the Aged Population

Objectives:
The overall purpose of the course is to update knowledge and skills necessary to assess, plan, implement, and evaluate quality nursing care for the aged

Implementation Plan:
A three-day workshop utilizing lecture, discussions, panels, audiovisuals, including videotaping of selected participant experiences and group work

Proposed Budget for the Project Period:
$4,500.00, including traineeships for students

Objectives:

Unit 1.   *Perspectives on Aging* (4½ hours)
         a. To update the nurse's knowledge of the aging process—biological, psychological, social, and socioeconomic
         b. To discuss the problems of the aging

Unit 2.   *Legislation* (2 hours)
         a. To update the participant's knowledge concerning federal and state legislation as it relates to regulations which affect nursing homes and its impact on the provision of nursing care in the nursing home and home care settings

Unit 3.   *Medications* (2 hours)
         a. To familiarize the participant with major medications administered to the aged
         b. To make the participant aware of medication side effects.
         c. To make the participant aware of the interactions occurring among major medications

Unit 4.   *Nursing Process* (3½ hours)
         a. To update the nurse's knowledge of the assessment, planning, implementing, and evaluating of nursing care
         b. To develop an understanding of the standards of gerontological nursing practice and their application

Unit 5.   *Preservation and Restoration of Function* (3 hours)
         a. To update the nurse's knowledge of preventive care and restorative methods
         b. To consider the physical, psychological (emo-

tional), and environmental care in institutional and other environmental factors in long-term settings

Unit 6. *Staff Development* (2 hours)
   a. To develop an understanding of staff development
   b. To discuss programs and procedures involved in staff development

Unit 7. *Resources Available for Staff Development* (3 hours)
   a. To preview and discuss selected audiovisual and other materials suitable for various levels in staff development

Unit 8. *Certification in Gerontological Nursing* (2 hours)
   a. To provide historical background of certification in the American Nurses' Association
   b. To develop an understanding of the purpose and process of certification
   c. To discuss the value of certification for patients or clients, the nurse, and the nursing profession

Unit 9. *Reality Orientation* (3½ hours)
   a. To provide knowledge of reality orientation as it applies to the aged
   b. To develop skills needed in the application of reality orientation in the care of the aged

Unit 10. *Individual and Group Consultation* (1½ hours, optional)
   a. To provide an opportunity for those participants who have special problems to meet with individuals or groups of faculty for consultation

Course Description:

A. Course Content

Unit 1. *Perspectives on Aging*
   a. The aging process—biological, psychological, social, and socioeconomic
   b. The problems of aging—interpersonal relations, health, housing, retirement

Unit 2. *Legislation*
  a. The development of federal nursing home and home care regulations
  b. Interpretation of the federal nursing home and home care regulations
  c. Comparison of federal and state nursing home and home care regulations
  d. Panel discussion—"How One Meets the Certification Standards"
  e. Reaction Panel—"Problems Confronting the Nursing Home Provider in Meeting Certification Standards"

Unit 3. *Medications*
  a. Drugs commonly administered to the aged
  b. Side effects of drugs
  c. Drug interactions

Unit 4. *Nursing Process*
  a. Components of a nursing care plan
  b. Assessing an aged client's needs
  c. Making a nursing diagnosis
  d. Developing short- and long-term goals
  e. Selecting nursing interventions
  f. Evaluating nursing care

Unit 5. *Preservation and Restoration of Function*
  a. Principles of rehabilitation—preservation and restoration of function
  b. Nursing process as applied to rehabilitation
  c. Psychological impact
  d. Sociological implications

Unit 6. *Staff Development*
  a. Process of staff development
  b. Specific procedures and program features
  c. Implementation

Unit 7. *Resources Available for Staff Development*
  a. Audiovisual materials
  b. Books, pamphlets
  c. Materials
  d. Continuing education

A Short-term Training Program

Unit 8. *Certification*
    a. History
    b. Purpose
    c. Procedures
Unit 9. *Reality Orientation*
    a. Description
    b. Application to the elderly
    c. Exemplary programs
Unit 10. *Individual and Group Consultation* (optional)
    a. Discussion with faculty concerning special participant problems identified during workshop

B. Methods of teaching to be utilized:
Lecture, discussions, panels, audiovisuals, including videotaping of selected participant experiences and group work
C. Required nonclassroom training activities, if any:
Library resources will be made available for participants
D. Special training facilities required, if any:
None are required
E. Instructional Staff:
Janet L. Gelein, R.N., M.S.N.
Alice L. Gallagher, R.N., M.S.N.
Claudette V. Campbell, R.N., M.P.H.
Roseann Marsicano, R.N., B.S.
Robert G. Pietrusko, Pharm.
Joanne Ryan, R.N., M.N.
Sister Paul Gabriel Wilhere, R.N., M.Ed.
Laurie M. Gunter, R.N., Ph.D.
Lois K. Waters, R.N., Ed.D.
Catharine Kopac, B.S.N.
Dolores Jean Hanyak, R.N., M.S.N.
Thomas J. Jennings, Jr., M.Ed.
F. Total hours of course instruction
21½ hours of required course instruction
1½ hours of optional instruction
6½ hours minimum course offering during a day

WORKSHOP EVALUATION FORM*

Update (II) Knowledge and Skills of Registered Nurses Who Serve the Aged Population

PLEASE RETURN THE COMPLETED EVALUATION FORM BEFORE YOU LEAVE

The purposes of this questionnaire are: (a) to obtain basic demographic data about individuals who attended the Workshop; (b) to obtain your impressions about the relative success (or failure) of various activities in the Workshop; (c) to determine how effectively the Workshop met its stated objectives; and (d) to obtain your suggestions for future programs. Your opinions will be appreciated in helping us to evaluate the present Workshop and in planning future programs.

Place a check in the selection of your choice.

1. Employment in nursing
    a. ( ) Employed full time
    b. ( ) Employed part time
    c. ( ) Not employed
2. Field of employment
    a. ( ) Hospital
    b. ( ) Nursing Home
    c. ( ) School of Nursing
    d. ( ) Private Duty
    e. ( ) Public Health
    f. ( ) Other (Specify)
3. Type of Position
    a. ( ) Administrator
    b. ( ) Director
    c. ( ) Supervisor
    d. ( ) In-service Education
    e. ( ) Head Nurse

*The authors acknowledge the assistance of Thomas Jennings in the preparation of the evaluation form.

A Short-term Training Program

    f. ( ) General Staff
    g. ( ) Private Duty
    h. ( ) Faculty
    i. ( ) Public Health
    j. ( ) Other (Specify)
4. Practice Area
    a. ( ) Geriatric
    b. ( ) Gynecologic/Obstetric
    c. ( ) Medical/Surgical
    d. ( ) Pediatric/Maternal Child Health
    e. ( ) Psychiatric/Mental Health
    f. ( ) Public Health
    g. ( ) ICU-CCU
    h. ( ) Other (Specify)
5. Type of Licensure
    a. ( ) Registered Nurse
    b. ( ) Practical Nurse
    c. ( ) Other (Specify)
6. Conference topic
    a. ( ) Of much interest
    b. ( ) Of moderate interest
    c. ( ) Not interesting
7. Organization of conference
    a. ( ) Excellent
    b. ( ) Very good
    c. ( ) Good
    d. ( ) Poor
8. In evaluating the impact of the conference as a whole, approximately how much of the program was new information to you?
    a. ( ) None
    b. ( ) A little
    c. ( ) About half
    d. ( ) Most
    e. ( ) All new
9. In evaluating the impact of the conference as a whole, approximately how much improved understanding do you think you obtained as compared to what you had?

a. ( ) None
   b. ( ) A little
   c. ( ) Much
   d. ( ) All new
10. Please list additional topics you would have liked to discuss in this conference. (If you have no additional topics to suggest, please indicate by writing NONE.)

11. What topics do you think could have been eliminated from this conference? (If you think that no topics could have been eliminated from the conference, please indicate by writing NONE.)

12. What do you consider to be the *most desirable* aspects of the conference?

13. What suggestions, changes, modifications, etc., would you like to see made in the conference to improve its relevance, instructional impact, usefulness, etc.? (If you have no suggestions to make, please indicate by writing NONE.)

14. What kinds of topics would you like to see included in future conferences? (If you have no specific topics to request, please indicate by writing NONE.)

The following questions will help to determine how effectively the workshop has met specific objectives. Complete only those items which apply to sessions you attended. If not applicable, write "NOT ATTENDED" in the space provided.

1. List four ways in which the aging process affects an individual's life:
   (a)
   (b)
   (c)
   (d)
2. Provide one example each of the physical, social, and emotional problems experienced by the aged.
   (a) physical:
   (b) social:
   (c) emotional:
3. Give an example of recent legislative regulations which have an impact on the provision of nursing care in nursing homes or home care settings.

4. Select three major medications and complete the chart as indicated.

	Major Medications	Possible Side Effects	Medication Interactions
(a)			
(b)			
(c)			

5. What are the four steps of the nursing process?
   (a)
   (b)
   (c)
   (d)

6. Describe one underlying principle for each of the following:
   (a) Preservation of function:

   (b) Restoration of function:

7. Specify two components recommended for an effective staff development program.
   (a)
   (b)
8. Identify three types of sources appropriate for the aquisition of staff development materials:
   (a)
   (b)
   (c)
9. Briefly describe the purpose and process of certification in gerontological nursing.

10. List three skills needed in the application of reality orientation in the care of the aged.
    (a)
    (b)
    (c)

Please return the completed evaluation form before you leave. A box labelled "EVALUATIONS" will be provided for this purpose. Thank you.

Bibliography

Chapter 1 References

1. Bevan, William. "On Growing Old in America," *Science*, (September 8, 1972): 839.
2. Department of Health, Education and Welfare. *Policy Guidelines for Special Project Grants for Improvement in Nurse Training.* Bethesda, Md.: Bureau of Health Manpower Education, 1969.

Chapter 2 References

1. Green, Robert Montraeille. *A Translation of Galen's Hygiene.* Springfield, Ill.: Charles C Thomas, Publisher, 1951, p. 202.
2. Butler, Robert N. *Why Survive? Being Old In America.* New York: Harper and Row, Publishers, 1975, p. 496.
3. Butler, Robert N., and Lewis, Myrna I. *Aging and Mental Health: Positive Psychosocial Approaches.* St. Louis: The C. V. Mosby Company, 1973.
4. Brubaker, Timothy H., and Powers, Edward A. "The Stereotype of 'Old': A Review and Alternative Approach." *Journal of Gerontology* 31 (July 1976): 441–447.
5. Institute of Life Insurance and the Health Insurance Institute. *Family News and Features* (May 1976): 1.
6. Neugarten, Bernice L. "The Young-Old." *The University of Chicago Magazine*, 68 (Autumn 1975): 22–23.
7. Vivian, Valerie. "Report from the Congress on the Quality of Life—The Later Years." *Health Education* (July/August, 1975): 16–18.

8. Neugarten, pp. 22–23.
9. Butler, *Why Survive?*
10. Butler, Robert N. "Looking Forward to What? The Life Review, Legacy, and Excessive Identity," *American Behavioral Scientist*, 14 (September-October, 1970), 121–128.
11. Busse, Ewald W. "Geriatrics Today—An Overview," *American Journal of Psychiatry*, 123:10, (April, 1967): 1226–33.
12. Fuchs, Victor R. *Who Shall Live? Health Economics and Social Choice.* New York: Basic Books, Inc., 1975, p. 143.
13. Cohen, Elias. "Comment Editors Note," *The Gerontologist*, (May 1976): 270, 275.

Chapter 3 References

1. Birren, James E., and Clayton, Vivian. "History of Gerontology," in Diana S. Woodruff and James E. Birren (eds.), *Aging: Scientific Perspectives and Social Issues.* New York: Van Nostrand Company, 1975.
2. Davis, Barbara A. "Coming of Age: A Challenge for Geriatric Nursing," *Journal of the American Geriatric Society*, 16 (October, 1968): 1100–1106.
3. Davis, Barbara A. "Geriatric Nursing Through the Looking Glass," *The Journal of the New York State Nurses Association*, (Winter 1971): 7–12.
4. "From 70 to 21,563: Division of Geriatric Nursing Practice," *Nursing Outlook*, 16 (June, 1968): 19.
5. "Standards for Geriatric Nursing Practice," *The American Journal of Nursing*, 70 (September, 1970): 1894–1897.
6. Norton, Doreen. "Nursing in Geriatrics," *Gerontologia Clinica*, 7 (1965): 51–60.
7. Havighurst, Robert J. "A World View of Gerontology," in Clyde B. Vedder (ed.), *Gerontology, A Book of Readings.* Springfield, Ill.: Charles C Thomas Publisher, 1963, p. 21.
8. "Standards for Geriatric Nursing Practice," pp. 1894–1897.
9. Norton, pp. 51–60.
10. Abdellah, Faye, and Levine, Eugene. *Better Patient Care through Nursing Research.* New York: The Macmillan Company, 1965.

Chapter 4 References

1. American Nurses' Association. "Auxiliary Personnel in Nursing Service," *The American Journal of Nursing*, 62 (July, 1962): 72–73.

2. National League for Nursing, Department of Practical Nursing Programs, the Steering Committee. "Statement on Training for Health Occupations," *Nursing Outlook,* 10 (August, 1962): 542–543.
3. "Nurse's Aide as Aids to Nursing," *Nursing Outlook,* 10 (August, 1962): 505.
4. Schwab, Sister Marilyn. "Where Nurse's Aides Don't Do All the Nursing Care," *Journal of Gerontological Nursing,* 2 (May/June 1976): 20–23.

Chapter 4 Suggested Readings

Bartoo, Margaret A., and Schwind, Bernard. "Alaska's Rural Home Helper Program," *New Outlook for the Blind,* 66 (June, 1972): 167–168.

Bush, M. Laura. "Itinerant Inservice Educator," *Nursing Outlook,* 21 (January, 1973): 25–27.

Ettinger, Ann L. "What Aides Can Do in Day Care Centers," *American Journal of Nursing,* 70 (June, 1970): 1288–1291.

Friedman, Jacob H., and Spada, Assunta R. "A Psychiatric Training Program for High School Students Assigned to a Geriatric Service," *Mental Hygiene,* 54 (July, 1970): 427–429.

Gale, Charlotte B. "Walking in the Aide's Shoes," *American Journal of Nursing,* 73 (April, 1973): 628–631.

Gartner, Alan. *Paraprofessionals and Their Performance, A Survey of Education, Health, and Social Service Programs.* New York: Praeger Publishers, 1971, pp. 3–4, 67–68.

Hameister, Dennis R. "Competencies of Nurses' Aides and the Design of In-Service Education." Paper prepared for presentation at the annual meeting of the Gerontological Society, Portland, Oregon, October 29–November 1, 1974.

Hameister, Dennis R. "Nurses Aides In-Service Education–An Institutional Profile." Paper prepared for presentation at the annual meeting of the Gerontological Society, Louisville, Kentucky, October 26–30, 1975.

Ryan, Joanne E. *Partners in Health–The Aide and the Elderly.* (Mimeographed.) University Park, Pa: The Pennsylvania State University, 1976.

Stolten, Jane Henry. *The Geriatric Aide.* Boston: Little, Brown and Company, 1973.

Chapter 5 References

1. National League for Nursing. *Licensed Practical Nurses in Nursing Services.* Publication No. 38-1457. New York: National League for Nursing, 1972, Appendix 1, pp. 25–29.
2. The Practical Nurse Act, P. L. 1295, 1965; Amended January 13, 1966.
3. From the *Pennsylvania Bulletin*, 2 (September 9, 1972).

Chapter 6 References

1. U.S. Senate, Special Committee on Aging. *Research and Training in Gerontology.* Washington, D.C.: Government Printing Office, 1971.
2. U.S. Senate, Special Committee on Aging, Subcommittee on Long-term Care. *Nursing Home Care in the United States: Failure in Public Policy, Nurses in Nursing Homes: The Heavy Burden* (Supporting Paper No. 4). Washington, D.C.: Government Printing Office, 1975, p. 369.
3. Brown, E. L. *Nursing Reconsidered, a Study of Change* (Part I). Philadelphia: J. B. Lippincott Co., 1970, p. 202.
4. American Nurses' Association. *Nursing and Long-Term Care: Toward Quality Care for the Aging.* American Nurses' Association, 1975, pp. xv, 36.
5. Moses, D. V., and Lake, C. S. "Geriatrics in the Baccalaureate Nursing Curriculum," *Nursing Outlook,* 16 (July, 1968): 41–43.
6. U.S. Senate, Special Committee on Aging, Subcommittee on Long-term Care, p. 369.
7. Burnside, I. M. *Nursing and the Aged.* New York: McGraw-Hill Book Co., 1975.
8. Browning, M. H. (comp.). *Nursing and the Aging Patient.* New York: American Journal of Nursing Co., 1974.
9. Gunter, L. M. "A New Look at the Older Patient in the Community," *Nursing Forum,* 8 (1969): 50–63.
10. Brown, M. I. "Nursing of the Aging and Aged," in A. B. Chin (ed.), *Working with Older People* (Vol. IV), Clinical Aspects of Aging. Washington, D.C.: Government Printing Office, 1971.
11. Gagne, R., and Briggs, L. J. *Principles of Instructional Design.* New York: Holt, Rhinehart and Winston, 1974.
12. Moses and Lake, pp. 41–43.
13. Rothkopf, E. Z. "The Concept of Mathemagenic Activities," *Review of Educational Research,* 40 (June 1970): 325–334.

Chapter 7 References

1. Kushner, Rose E., and Bunch, Marion E. (eds.). *Graduate Education in Aging Within the Social Sciences.* Ann Arbor, Mich: Division of Gerontology, The University of Michigan, 1967.
2. National League for Nursing, Department of Baccalaureate and Higher Degree Programs. *Criteria for the Appraisal of Baccalaureate and Higher Degree Programs in Nursing.* New York: National League for Nursing, 1972.
3. National League for Nursing. *Policies and Procedures of Accreditation for Programs in Nursing Education.* New York: National League for Nursing, 1976.
4. The Council of Graduate Schools in the United States. *The Master's Degree.* Washington, D.C.: Council of Graduate Schools in the United States (no date).
5. Gaff, Jerry G., and Wilson, Robert C. "The Teaching Environment," *American Association of University Professors Bulletin,* 57 (December, 1971): 475–493.
6. Dimond, E. Grey. "A Safe Physician," *Tempo,* 3 (Fall, 1971): 7–9.
7. Nayapadi, T. J. "The Qualities of Nursing," *Nursing Mirror,* 140 (April 17, 1975): 65–67.
8. Caldwell, E., and Hegner, B. *Geriatrics, A Study of Maturity.* Albany: Delwar Publishers, 1975, p. 24.
9. Hodkinson, M. A. "Future of Geriatric Nursing," *Nursing Mirror and Midwives Journal,* 113 (January 12, 1962): iii–v.
10. Felton, Geraldene. "Socialization and Graduate Education in Nursing: Exploration in Strategy," *Journal, N.Y.S.N.A.,* (New York State Nurses Association), 5, Convention Papers, 15–22.
11. Committee on Standards for Geriatric Nursing Practice. "Standards for Geriatric Nursing Practice," *American Journal of Nursing,* 70 (September, 1970): 1894–1897.
12. American Nurses' Association. *Standards for Gerontological Nursing Practice,* Kansas City, Mo.: The American Nurses' Association, Inc., 1976.
13. Task Force on the Expanding Role of the Geriatric Nurse. *Guidelines for Short-term Continuing Education Programs Preparing the Geriatric Nurse Practitioner,* Kansas City, Mo.: The American Nurses' Association, Inc. 1974.
14. "Extending the Scope of Nursing Practice," *Nursing Outlook,* 20 (January, 1972): 46–52.
15. Norton, Doreen. "Nursing Geriatrics," *Gerontologia Clinica,* 7 (1965): 51–60.

16. "Extending the Scope of Nursing Practice," pp. 46–52.
17. Ibid.
18. Ibid.
19. Ibid.
20. Dr. Joseph D. Matarazzo in *Future Directions of Doctoral Education for Nurses.* Conference Report, Bethesda, Md.: Department of Health, Education and Welfare, Division of Nursing, 1971.

Chapter 7 Suggested Readings

Journals
Advances in Gerontological Research
Aging
Educational Gerontology
Experimental Aging Research
Experimental Gerontology
Geriatric Focus
Geriatrics
Gerontologia
Gerontologia Clinica
Gerontologist
Industrial Gerontology
Interdisciplinary Topics in Gerontology
International Journal of Aging and Human Development
Journal of the American Geriatrics Society
Journal of Geriatric Psychiatry
Journal of Gerontological Nursing
Journal of Gerontology
Mechanisms of Aging and Development

Indexes, Abstracts, Bibliographies
Excerpta Medica Foundation, *Excerpta Medica. Section 20. Gerontology and Geriatrics.* 1, 1958– .
Shock, Nathan W. *A Classified Bibliography of Gerontology and Geriatrics.* Stanford: Stanford University Press, 1957, 1963.
Shock, Nathan W. *Current Publications in Gerontology and Geriatrics.* 1962+ .
U.S. National Library of Medicine. *Index Medicus.* Monthly, annual cumulation. 1960– . Under various names this listing of medical literature covers 1879 to present.

Bibliography

Catalogue of the Ethel Percy Andrus Geontology Center. Vol. 1, author-title catalogue; Vol. 2, subject catalogue. Los Angeles: University of Southern California, 1976.

Schaie, K. W., and Zelinski, E. (comp.). *Intellectual Functioning and Aging: A Selected Bibliography.* Ethel Percy Andrus Gerontology Center. Los Angeles: University of Southern California, 1975.

A Selected, Annotated Bibliography on Aging and the Aged: 1968–1972. Council of Planning Libraries, Exchange Bibliography #319. Monticello, Ill., 1972.

National Council on the Aging. *Current Literature on Aging.* New York, 1957–

Words on Aging. A bibliography of selected annotated references compiled for the Administration on Aging by the Department of Health, Education and Welfare Library. Washington, D.C.: Government Printing Office, 1974. (3rd Printing.)

Aging in the Modern World. An annotated bibliography compiled for the U.S. Office of Aging by the Department of Health, Education and Welfare Library. Washington, D.C.: Government Printing Office, 1963.

Facts on Aging. Washington, D.C.: Government Printing Office, 1963– (irregular).

U.S. Public Health Service. *Nursing Care of the Aged.* An annotated bibliography for nurses. Public Health Service Publication No. 1603. Washington, D.C.: Government Printing Office, 1967.

Other References

The Handbooks of Aging Series. 3 Vol. James E. Birren, Editor-in-Chief. New York: Van Nostrand Reinhold, 1976.

Textbooks

Anderson, Helen C *Newton's Geriatric Nursing.* St. Louis: The C. V. Mosby Company, 1971.

Cowdry, S. V., and Steinberg, F. U. *The Care of the Geriatric Patient.* St. Louis: the C. V. Mosby Co., 1971.

Rossman, Isadore (ed.). *Clinical Geriatrics.* Philadelphia: J. B. Lippincott Co., 1971.

Chapter 8 References

1. Brown, Esther Lucille. *Nursing for the Future.* A report prepared for the Nursing Council. New York: Russell Sage Foundation, 1948.

2. Silver, Henry K., Ford, Loretta, C., and Day, Lewis R. "The Pediatric Nurse Practitioner Program: Expanding the Role of the Nurse to Provide Increased Health Care for Children," *Journal of the American Medical Association*, 204 (April 22, 1968): 298–302.
3. Stead, Eugene A., Jr. "Conserving Costly Talents—Providing Physicians New Assistants," *Journal of the American Medical Association*, 198 (December 5, 1966): 182–183.
4. Smith, Richard. "Medex," *Journal of the American Medical Association*, 211 (March 16, 1970): 1843–1845.
5. "AMA Urges Major New Roles for Nurses," *American Medical News*, 13 (February, 1970): 1, 8.
6. "The National Center for Health Services Research and Development." *Nursing Outlook*, 20 (January, 1972): 29.
7. "Definition: Nurse Practitioner, Nurse Clinician and Clinical Nurse Specialist." Mimeographed statement by the Congress for Nursing Practice, American Nurses' Association. Kansas City, Mo.: American Nurses' Association, May 8, 1974.
8. "Nurse Practitioner Training, Part II," *Federal Register*, 41 (January 23, 1976): 3555.
9. American Nurses' Association, Division on Geriatric Nursing Practice. *Guidelines for Short-Term Continuing Education Programs Preparing the Geriatric Nurse Practitioner.* Kansas City, Mo.: American Nurses' Association, 1974, p. 3.
10. "Extending the Scope of Nursing Practice." *Nursing Outlook*, 20 (January, 1972): 46–52.
11. *Federal Register*, p. 3555.
12. ANA Division on Geriatric Nursing Practice, p. 3.
13. Aradine, Carolyn R. "The Challenge of Clinical Nursing Practice in an Interdisciplinary Office Setting," *Nursing Forum*, 12 (1973): 291–302.
14. Bessman, Alice N. "Comparison of Medical Care in Nurse Clinician and Physician Clinics in Medical School Affiliated Hospitals," *Journal of Chronic Disease*, 27 (March, 1974): 115–125.
15. Chappell, James A., and Drogos, Patricia A. "Evaluation of Infant Care by a Nurse Practitioner," *Pediatrics*, 49 (June, 1972): 871–877.
16. Charney, Evan, and Kitzman, Harriet. "The Child-Health Nurse (Pediatric Nurse Practitioner) in Private Practice: A Controlled Trial," *New England Journal of Medicine*, 285 (December, 9, 1971): 1353–1358.
17. Duncan, B., Smith, A. N., and Silver, H. K. "Comparison of the Physical Assessment of Children by Pediatric Nurse Practitioners

and Pediatricians," *American Journal of Public Health,* 61 (June, 1971): 1170–1176.
18. Flynn, Beverly C. "The Effectiveness of Nurse Clinicians Service Delivery," *American Journal of Public Health,* 64 (June, 1974): 604–611.
19. Yankauer, A., Tripp, S., Andrews, P., and Connelly, John P. "The Outcomes and Service Input of a Pediatric Nurse Practitioner Training Program—Nurse Practitioner Training Outcomes," *American Journal of Public Health,* 62 (March, 1972): 347–353.
20. Heppler, Jacqueline. "Gerontological Nurse Practitioner: Change Agents in the Health Care Delivery Systems for the Aged," *Journal of Gerontological Nursing,* 2 (May–June, 1976): 38–40.
21. Anderson, Eva, Cooley, Elaine, and Sparrow, Alma. "Role and Preparation of the Adult/Geriatric Nurse Associate," *Minnesota Medicine* (October, 1973): 69–72.
22. Brower, Terri F., Bedgio, Donna, Baker, Brydie J., and Tharp, Terril S. "The Geriatric Nurse Practitioner: An Expanded Role for the Care of the Older Adult," *Journal of Gerontological Nursing,* 2 (July–August, 1976): 17–20.
23. "Extending the Scope of Nursing Practice," pp. 46–52.
24. *HEW News.* Department of Health, Education and Welfare, December 20, 1976.
25. *HEW News.*

Chapter 9 References

1. Kelly, Lucie Young. *Dimensions of Professional Nursing.* 3rd ed. New York: Macmillan Publishing Co., 1975, pp. 107–09.
2. American Nurses' Association. *Continuing Education in Nursing Guidelines for State Voluntary and Mandatory Systems.* Kansas City, Mo.: American Nurses' Association, 1975, pp. 22–24.
3. American Nurses' Association. *Code for Nurses With Interpretive Statements.* Kansas City, Mo.: American Nurses' Association, 1976.
4. Kubat, Janice. "Correlates of Professional Obsolescence: Part I," *The Journal of Continuing Education in Nursing,* 6 (November–December 1975): 22–29.
5. Tobin, Helen M., Yoder, Pat S., Hull, Peggy K., and Scott, Barbara Clark. *The Process of Staff Development,* St. Louis: The C. V. Mosby Company, 1974, pp. 28–30.
6. American Nurses' Association. *Standards for Gerontological Nursing Practice.* Kansas City, Mo.: American Nurses' Association, 1976.

7. American Nurses' Association. *Guidelines for Short-Term Continuing Education Programs Preparing the Geriatric Nurse Practitioner.* Kansas City, Mo.: American Nurses' Association, 1974.
8. American Nurses' Association. *Geriatric Nursing Certification.* Kansas City, Mo.: American Nurses' Association, 1973.
9. National League for Nursing. *Understanding the Aging Process and the Institutionalized Elderly Person: An Instructor's Guide.* Publication No. 38-1616. New York: National League for Nursing, 1976.
10. National League for Nursing. *Understanding the Aging Process and the Institutionalized Elderly Person: An Instruction Program,* Publication No. 38-1615. New York: National League for Nursing, 1976.
11. Tobin et al.
12. Fatula, Betty J. "Facilitating Adult Learning." (Mimeograph.) University Park, Pa.: Gerontology Center, Institute for the Study of Human Development, January, 1977.
13. Rakowski, William R. "Facilitating Discussion Groups." (Mimeograph.) University Park, Pa.: Gerontology Center, Institute for the Study of Human Development, January, 1977.
14. Mayne, Marion S., *A Guide to Inservice Education for Nursing Personnel in Nursing Homes.* Los Angeles, Calif.: U.C.L.A. Extension, 1971.
15. Fatula.
16. Hickey, Tom, and Fatula, Betty. *Gerontology Practitioner Training Manual: Sensory Deprivation and the Elderly.* Vol. I. University Park, Pa: The Pennsylvania State University, 1976.
17. Zerbe, Melissa, and Hickey, Tom. *Gerontology Practitioner Training Manual: Self-Maintenance Skills for the Elderly.* Vol. II. University Park, Pa.: The Pennsylvania State University, 1976.
18. Greenberg, Lois, Fatula, Betty, Hameister, Dennis R., and Hickey, Tom. *Gerontology Practitioner Training Manual: Communication Skills in the Gerontological Environment.* Vol. III. University Park, Pa.: The Pennsylvania State University, 1976.
19. Hickey, Tom, Axinn, Paul, Fatula, Betty, and Hameister, Dennis R. *Gerontology Practitioner Training Manual: Loss Reaction and Grief Management.* Vol. IV. University Park, Pa.: The Pennsylvania State University, 1976.
20. Kelly, p. 107.
21. Tobin et al., pp. 28–30.

Bibliography

Appendix B Reference

1. Anderson, T., et al., "A Computer-based Study Management System," *Educational Psychologist*, 11 (1974): 36–45.

Appendix D Reference

1. Public Health Traineeship Program. *Traineeship Grants for Short-Term Training (Section 306, PHS Act)*. DHEW Publication No. (HRA) 75-45. Bethesda, Md.: Department of Health, Education and Welfare, 1975, p. 1.

Index

Administration of graduate programs. *See* Organization of graduate programs
Administrator of graduate programs in gerontic nursing, 90
Age
 as determinant of nursing needs, 32
 as index to client characteristics, 32
Aged, the
 health care delivery for, 16
 health care needs of, 2
 healthy, 2, 12
 institutional care of, 2, 12
 numbers of, 16, 67
Aging
 as a normal process, 12, 58
 process of, 20–22
American Nurses' Association
 Committee on Standards for Geriatric Nursing Practice, 29, 30
 Congress for Nursing Practice, 141
 definition of geriatric nursing, 36
 Division of Geriatric Nursing Practice, 28, 66, 67
 Division of Gerontological Nursing Practice, 30
 guidelines for voluntary and mandatory continuing education systems, 148
 Report from the Committee on Skilled Nursing Care, 66
 Standards for Continuing Education, 148
 Standards of Nursing Practice, 92
Attitudes toward the aged, 18, 67, 68

Baccalaureate degree programs
 arguments supporting instruction in gerontics in, 67–68
 geriatric nursing courses in, 66
 importance of geriatric programs in, 67–69
 outline for introductory course in gerontic nursing in, 73–76

Clinical teaching setting for gerontics courses
 guidelines for protecting patients in, 92–93

205

Clinical teaching (*continued*)
  incidence reports in, 92–93
  legal status of student in, 92
  responsibility for negligent acts in, 93
  use of standards of practice in, 92
Competencies expected at master's level
  in health nursing, 107–108
  for the long-term care nurse, 109–111
  for the nurse administrator of long-term care facilities, 111
  for the nurse educator, 111–112
  for the primary care nurse, 108–109
Composite educational program for geriatric nursing
  content in aging, 6–9
  educational mechanisms in, 6–10
  educational materials for, 4–5
  guidelines for developing instructional units, 12
  guides to program development, 5–12
  levels of personnel to be taught, 3–4, 6–10
  objectives of, 3–4
  plans for (table), 6–11
Computer-managed review and examination in nursing care of the elderly, 170–179
Congress on the Quality of Life—the Later Years, 19–20
Continuing education. *See* Education, continuing

Council of Graduate Schools in the U.S., 87
Course model for computer-based instruction, 169–170
Course outline for gerontic nursing, 181–182
Courses, gerontological, 53
Courses in graduate curriculum
  areas covered, 123
  emphasis in, 123, 124
  examples of course outlines, 124–128, 128–133
  in nursing specializations, 128–133
Curriculum designs
  for continuing education programs for LPNs, 55–61
  for on-the-job training courses for nurse's aides, 45–52

Decrements in the elderly, 34–35
Division of Geriatric Nursing Practice of the ANA, 12, 28, 66, 67, 89, 102
Doctoral programs, curriculum framework for, 112–114

Education
  basic nursing, 81
  gerontic nursing, 65–79
  inservice, 148
Education, continuing
  for aides, 150–151
  ANA guidelines for, 148–149
  content of courses in, 153–156
  current issues in, 160–162
  format for programs in, 156–160
  for gerontic nurse specialist, 152
  for gerontic nursing, 147–164

Guidelines for Short-Term Continuing Education Programs Preparing the Geriatric Nurse Practitioner, 143
  identification of needs for, 154–156
  length of programs in, 145
  for nurse gerontologist, 152–153
  problems in, 144–145
  programs for, 54, 144
  recommendations for, 163–165
  for RNs, 13, 54, 151–152
  training modules for, 159–160
Education in gerontic nursing, undergraduate
  arguments for developing curriculum in, 67–68
  arguments supporting need for, 69–70
  course outline for, 73–76
  courses in, 66
  curriculums for, 70–73
  expected competencies of students, 72–73
  instructional content, 73–76
  instructional means, 77
  measurement of instruction outcomes, 77–79
  need for, 65
  teachability of subject matter, 69
Emotions expressed by the aged, 18
Environmental deprivation, influence on the aged of, 2, 12
Evaluation of graduate programs, 136–138
  by the graduate school faculty, 137
  by the National League for Nursing, 137
  by review of theses, 137–138
Examples of graduate programs and courses. *See* Pennsylvania State University
Expertise in nursing care of the aging, 65–67

Facilities and space for programs in gerontic nursing, 91–92
Faculty for graduate programs
  budgetary provisions for, 99
  clinical teaching, implications of, 93, 94
  determining needs, 93–94
  expected activities of, 94–95
  joint appointments, 96, 97, 98
  preceptors or docents, 97
  preparation of, 94
  relationship to service personnel, 96, 98–99
  shortage of, 94
  teaching functions of nursing service personnel, 97
Family relationships and the elderly, 20
Framework for graduate programs, 102–111

Geriatric nurse, desirable qualities of, 99
Geriatric nurse practitioner
  defined, 140, 141
  Guidelines for Short-Term Continuing Education Programs Preparing the Geriatric Nurse Practitioner, 143
  preparation of, 139–146
  problems and issues concerning, 143–144

Geriatric nursing
  ANA Division of Geriatric Nursing Practice, 28
  concerns of, 29
  definition of, 29, 30, 36
  system of certification for practice, 66
  See also Composite educational program for geriatric nursing
Geriatrics, definition of, 29–30, 36
Gerontic nurse
  concerns of, 37
  need for, 28
Gerontic nursing
  definition of, 30–35
  graduate education for. *See* Graduate education in nursing
Gerontologic nursing, 30, 31
Gerontology
  as an applied science, 35
  basic concepts of, 27
  courses in, 53
  definition of, 35
  medical, 35–36
  nursing, 35, 37, 38
  science of, 15, 35, 37
  social, 35–36
Graduate education in nursing
  academic objectives of, 83
  courses in the curriculum, 114
  curriculum framework for doctoral programs, 112–114
  evaluation of programs, 136–138
  examples of programs and courses, 114–123
  framework for, 102–112
  issues in, 89–90
  nature of, 82
  organization of programs for, 90–102
  planning programs for, 87–89
  preceptor relationship in, 100–101
  professional objectives of, 83–84
  professional socialization in, 100, 101
  purpose of programs in, 82
  seminar, use of, 133–136
  specialization courses in, 128–133
  as a specialty, 28
  See also Pennsylvania State University
Guidelines for nurse practitioner programs, 142–143
Guide to Content Analysis for Computer-Based Nursing Courses (table), 165–176

Health care for the aging
  access to, 23
  costs of, 23
  Medicaid, 23
  Medicare, 23
Health and disease in the aging, 22–23
Health nursing, 107–108
  competencies expected at the master's level, 108–109
Health, Education and Welfare, Committee to Study Extended Roles for Nurses, 103, 142, 144
Health and Manpower Act of 1968, 3
Health Resources Administration, Bureau of Health Man-

power, Division of Nursing, 99
Heredity and the aging process, 22

Income, distribution of, 6, 19
Independence of the elderly, 20
Inservice education, 13, 55
Institutionalization of the aged, 2, 20, 24–25
  alternatives to, 24–25
  quality of, 1
Isolation of the aged, 19
Issues in care of the aging
  alternatives to institutional care, 24–25
  distribution of income, 19
  health and disease, 22–23
  myths about the aged, 18
  old age and cultural values, 23–25
  old age and our society, 16–20
  old age as a stage in development, 20–23
  professional caretakers, 24
  self-actualization, 21–22
  stereotypes of the aged, 16, 17, 18, 19, 20, 33
  support systems, 19–20
Issues in continuing education
  effectiveness of programs, 161
  evaluation of programs, 162
  kinds of education needed, 162
  mandatory requirement for relicensure, 160–161
Issues in graduate education
  types of degrees, 89
  career goals of students, 89
  titles for specialists, 89
  emphasis of programs, 89

Journal of Continuing Education, 157
Journal of Gerontological Nursing, 103

Life expectancy, 1, 16
Licensed Practical Nurse
  continuing education programs for, 57
  curriculum design for inservice and continuing education, 55–57
  expected competencies for, 57
  modules for continuing education program, 58–63
  NLN statement of functions and qualifications for, 53
  preparation for gerontic nursing, 53–63
Living arrangements for the aging, 20
Long-term care nursing
  example of course in, 131–133
  expected competencies of nursing administrator in, 112
  expected competencies of nurses in, 131–133
Losses, effects on the aged, 17

Master of Nursing degree, 84–85, 115
Master of Science degree, 84, 85–86, 115, 120–123
Misconceptions about aging, 20
Myths about aging, 17–18
  chronological measurements of age, 18
  disengagement, 18

Myths about aging (*continued*)
  inflexibility, 18
  senility, 18
  serenity, 18
  unproductivity, 18

National Institute of Mental Health and Drug Abuse, 99
National League for Nursing
  Criteria for the Appraisal of Baccalaureate and Higher Degree Programs in Nursing, 87
  Department of Baccalaureate and Higher Degree Programs, 87
  Department of Practical Nursing Programs, 87
  Training for Health Occupations, 41
Norton, Doreen, 29, 30, 36, 103
Nurse administrator, 111
Nurse educator, 111–112
Nurse practitioner, 3, 83, 139–146
  concerns of, 141
  definition of, 141
  educational preparation, 83, 139–146
  numbers needed, 144
  problems and issues concerning, 143–144
  qualifications for, 141
  role of, 144
  salaries of, 144, 146
  See also Programs for nurse practitioners
Nurse Training Act of 1971, 3
Nurse Training Act of 1975, 142
Nurse's aide, 13, 41–52, 150, 151
Nursing the aged
  geriatric nursing, 36–37
  gerontic nursing, 30–35
  gerontological nursing, 35–36
  historical perspectives, 27–30
  interactions of research and practice in, 37
Nursing homes, 1, 2, 27, 28
Nursing specialization courses
  clinical process in health care and nursing, 128–129
  health nursing, 129–130
  long-term care nursing, 131–132
  primary care nursing, 130–131
  seminar, 133
  See also Pennsylvania State University

Objectives of graduate programs, 83–87
Objectives for Older Americans, 25–26
Old age
  attitudes toward, 17
  and cultural values, 23–25
  emotional reactions in, 18
  life-span approach to, 89
  and our society, 16–20
  problem-centered approach to, 89
  quality of life in, 16, 17
  stereotypes of, 16, 17, 18, 20
  as a tragedy, 17
Older Americans Act, 25–26
On-the-job training program for the nurse's aide
  course content for, 46–52
  description of, 45
  length of, 45
  objectives of, 46
  prerequisites for, 45
  program outline for, 46–52

Index

Organization of graduate programs
 administration, 90
 facilities for, 91–92
 faculty for, 93–99
 setting for clinical teaching, 92
 students in, 99–102

Pennsylvania State University graduate courses and programs in nursing, 115–138
 courses in nursing specialization, 128–133
 Master of Nursing degree, 115
 Master of Science degree, 115
 Master of Science with preparation for gerontic nursing, 120–123
 outlines of courses in the graduate curriculum, 124–128
 program with a specialization in health nursing and clinical option in adult health and aging, 116–120
Primary care for the elderly, 141, 142
Primary care nursing
 defined, 108
 example of course in, 130–131
 nurse competencies expected in, 108–109
Primex, 140
Programs for nurse practitioners
 costs of, 145–146
 federal grants for, 142
 Guidelines for short-term continuing education programs preparing the geriatric nurse practitioner, 143
 variations in length of, 144

Proposal to establish a graduate program in gerontic nursing, how to prepare, 88–89

Quality of life for the aged, 16, 17, 58–59

Recommendations
 for continuing education for gerontic nurses, 162–164
 for gerontic nursing education, 13–14
Research, nursing
 interaction with practice, 37
 nursing gerontology and, 36–37
Review and examination of course in care of the elderly, 170–179

Self-actualization, 21–22
Self-perception, 21
Seminar
 brief outline for, 134–135
 evaluation of, 134
 examples of course outline for, 133–136
Senate Subcommittee on Long-Term Care, 66
Senility, 18
Serenity, errors in the myth, 18
Short-term continuing education training programs, sample, 183–191
Social Security Act, 27
Specialists, need for, 141–142
Specialization in health nursing
 example of program for, 116–120
 need for, at graduate level, 14
 purpose of, 116

Stereotypes of the aged, 16, 17, 18, 19, 20, 33
Students
  baccalaureate, 2
  graduate assistantships for, 101
  in graduate programs, 99–102
  important qualities of, 99–100
  preceptor relationship, 101
  professional socialization, 101
Support systems for the aged, 16

Training program for nurse's aide
  course content, 46
  description of, 45
  length of, 45
  objectives of, 46
  program outline for, 46–52

Undergraduate education in gerontic nursing. *See* Education in gerontic nursing, undergraduate
U.S. Senate Special Committee on Aging, report on deficiency in training of care for the aged, 65–66